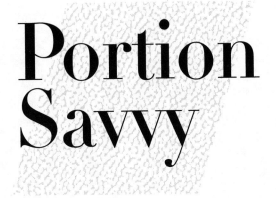

Portion Savvy

Portion Savvy

THE 30-DAY SMART PLAN FOR EATING WELL

Carrie Latt Wiatt, M.S.,

WITH Elizabeth Miles

POCKET BOOKS
New York London Toronto Sydney Toyko Singapore

POCKET BOOKS, a division of Simon & Schuster Inc.
1230 Avenue of the Americas, New York, NY 10020

Copyright © 1999 by Carrie Latt Wiatt

All rights reserved, including the right to reproduce this book or portions thereof in any form whatsoever. For information address Pocket Books, 1230 Avenue of the Americas, New York, NY 10020

Library of Congress Cataloging-in-Publication Data

Wiatt, Carrie Latt.
Portion savvy : the 30-day smart plan for eating well / Carrie Latt Wiatt, with Elizabeth Miles.
p. cm.
Includes index.
ISBN 0-671-02416-7
1. Weight loss. 2. Food portions. 3. Reducing diets. I. Miles, Elizabeth. II. Title.
RM222.2.W4523 1999
613.2'5—dc21 98-41929

First Pocket Books hardcover printing January 1999

10 9 8 7 6 5 4 3 2 1

POCKET and colophon are registered trademarks of Simon & Schuster Inc.

Designed by Joseph Rutt
Interior photos by Rachel Latt

Printed in the U.S.A.

QF/✠/NMSG

To my nephew, Spencer

CONTENTS

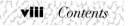

Portion savvy pop-outs follow page 78.

INTRODUCTION
RECONDITIONING THE AMERICAN APPETITE

A chic and cosmopolitan woman came to me after gaining ten pounds immediately upon moving to the United States from Brazil. Though she had lived in many countries, Sonia had never experienced a weight gain like this before.

"It's the portions they serve you here," she told me. "They're simply amazing. Somehow, without thinking, you manage to eat it all—then your stomach stretches, you start to expect all that food, and before you know it you're fat with a whole new set of eating habits!"

Poor Sonia. The customs officers had failed to warn her about the overfeeding of America.

No country in the world eats as much as we do or struggles so with weight problems and the attendant high rates of life-threatening disease. Overeating has become a dangerous epidemic. We can't rely on the food-pushers in the food industry or on the social structures of an overindulgent culture to save us from this catastrophe. We have to save ourselves.

Americans are deeply conditioned to overeat. From birth onward, we're presented with servings of food far in excess of our actual needs—at home, in restaurants, at the sandwich counter and the supermarket. Compounding the problem is scientific evidence that it's perfectly natural for animals confronted with abundant food to eat themselves silly. The result is that the blueprint we carry around in our minds for how much is enough is wrong.

We may live in the land of the free, but our culture has come to be characterized by complete lack of control. The dark underbelly of the American dream is the drive to acquire to the point of excess, and this culture of consumption has rubbed off on our eating habits. Just as having too many material goods can rob each one of its meaning, eating too much can erode our ability to derive pleasure and satisfaction from food. Overeating works like a drug in the body, numbing us to our feelings and preventing us from facing that profound, self-defining question: *How much is enough?*

Most people reading this book have probably been trained to overeat, and the first thing I want to say is, *overeating is not your fault.* It's simply the continuation of a historical trend, begun at the beginning of the twentieth century, in which affluence, a sedentary lifestyle, and lack of nutritional understanding have combined to create the American eating paradigm that more is better.

The facts in this book clearly prove this paradigm to be false. When it comes to the food you put in your body, the true paradigm is, *enough is enough.* Excess energy intake stresses out your system at every level—and though we now have the medical technology to live longer than ever before, we won't be able to unless we stop this killer habit. All the stress management in the world can't save you if you continue to stress your body with too much food.

As a nation, we've lost control—and the statistics show that it's getting worse every day. At this rate, we'll meet the new millennium devastated by nutritional disease. If we are to realize our potential and create a safe environment for our children, we must stop allowing ourselves to be victims of the food-pushers. We must find a new path to healthy bodies and minds.

I think I've been a nutritionist in my heart since I was a little girl growing up in a household without any boundaries or guidance on the topic of food. I was raised eating the same packaged and processed junk that everyone else did in the 1960s. I watched my mother lose and regain the same twenty pounds over and over on the crazy yo-yo diets that women used as feeble weapons against the fattening American diet. A strong personal conviction drove me to start cooking healthy food at a young age and ultimately to pursue a bachelor of science and master's degree in nutrition and food science.

I've been a nutritionist in professional practice for fifteen years, serving a broad range of clients with my Los Angeles company Diet Designs. The weight loss and management program I've created has attracted a high-profile clientele, including many movie stars. I founded Diet Designs to provide people with the tools they need to rebalance, recondition, escape the epidemic of overweight and establish a joyful new relationship with food, and unite mind and body in the creation of new habits that promise a longer, healthier, and higher-quality life.

And I've written *Portion Savvy* to recondition the American appetite.

WHAT IS PORTION SAVVY?

At Diet Designs, I'm part scientist, part therapist, part gourmet low-fat chef—but primarily I'm an educator. By teaching my clients the all-important basics of how to match their food intake to their energy needs, I enable them to achieve and maintain their best weight. I call all of the knowledge that goes into this seemingly simple but deceptively complex skill *portion savvy,* and with this book I've distilled that entire learning process into a monthlong plan you can do for yourself.

Portion savvy is a thirty-day learning program that gives you:

➤ The portion savvy and habits you need to achieve and maintain a healthy weight for a lifetime.
➤ The ability to consistently choose proven right-size portions for your energy needs and optimal weight.
➤ A set of visual/spatial, analytic/mathematical, and kinesthetic/sensory skills pertaining to food.
➤ A recipe collection of tantalizing low-fat dishes from Polenta Lasagna to Ginger-Crusted Salmon and Chocolate-Orange Biscotti, complete with detailed portioning instructions.

➤ The missing element in the lower-fat diet trends that have Americans eating less fat but consuming more calories and weighing more than ever before.

➤ A mind and body "click-in" that makes food management natural.

Becoming portion savvy is like learning to read. Once you have the skill, you possess an invaluable tool for life. And like reading, this skill makes everything easier.

THE ABCs OF EATING

What could initially seem more mysterious than moving your eyes over squiggly lines and making sense of them? And what, now that you know how to read, could be more automatic, necessary, and often fun? I kid my clients that most Americans are at the kindergarten level when it comes to knowing how much to eat—and just as words on a page were inscrutable at that age, portion savvy might seem complicated at the beginning. Soon, it will be automatic, and it will change your life forever.

Most people's eating habits are rooted in childhood and a distorted image of how much food is wanted or needed by the human body. Research has found that eating habits are notoriously hard to change—especially permanently.[1] You may already know that from your personal experience.

But psychologists have found that the same behavioral mechanisms that underlie bad habits also underlie good ones—and that *learning* can change *behavior.*

Portion savvy is a learning and behavior modification program based on tested psychological data and the experience of my own practice. It will help you replace your overfeeding habits with healthy ones. It's a hands-on, interactive learning experience designed to activate the feedback loop that links three things: the physical action of portioning food, the mental effort of encoding and remembering your servings, and the psychological pleasure of feeling satisfied. You'll cross-link your cognition and behavior to turn desire into action and action into results. In other words, you'll learn how to derive pleasure from right-size portions.

Many of my clients tell me that they receive their most powerful lesson at Diet Designs when they first see their right-size portions. Most people don't have any idea what a serving sized to their energy needs even *looks* like. At Diet Designs, I reeducate people's eyes by cooking and portioning their food for them; in this book, I've provided an equally powerful visual tool in the form of the portion savvy pop-outs: actual-size silhouettes that help you literally see a serving. Seeing is believing, and this is one of the ways in which you'll learn how much is enough for you.

Becoming portion savvy will enable you to redesign the food blueprint in your mind, then learn to remember it anytime, anywhere, the way you remember essential life truths and the sound of your mother's voice. Portion savvy will become a sixth sense, as natural as seeing and feeling.

MAGICAL MATH

Behind the smoke and mirrors of every successful diet is calorie restriction. I'm bluntly honest with my clients: The magic of my program's success isn't in pills or powders, but in forming two habits: *eating fewer calories* and *expending more calories.* It might not sound seductive, but it works and seems to be glamorous enough to count some of the country's most famous celebrities among its followers.

Burning fat is a mathematical process, and one of the reasons my clients love me is because I do the math that makes it happen on their behalf. Likewise, I've created the program in this book to take care of the numbers for you. There's no calorie-counting or calculators, nor are there required food combinations or forbidden nutrient groups.

In fact, becoming portion savvy isn't about "going on" a diet at all. It's about relearning your needs and how to satisfy them. It's an action plan to evolve your diet toward a healthier one. One step at a time, through small and attainable steps, you'll learn. You'll change. You'll shrink in circumference as you grow in understanding. Portion savvy involves physical and cognitive transformation.

Portion savvy people are never on or off a diet; instead, they have a portion savvy *mind-set.* They realize that every day is a diet—an individualized meal plan—no matter what they eat. By engaging in patterned behaviors, learning the nutritional facts, and fueling motivation to maximize potential, portion savvy people "click in" to this new mind-set that puts them on the fit track for good.

Mine is a mind-body approach that gives you the precious time you need to gradually acquire new habits, make mistakes and fix them, resize your eating blueprint to balance your energy equation, and do the deep subconscious work that leads to the magic moment of click-in. Everybody wants to start fast, but nobody wants to suffer, so over years in practice I've learned to pace my program at the speed of the subconscious mind. Savvy starts where thought begins, deep in the mind with images and dreams.

Just as negative addictions sneak up on us one day at a time, so do positive habits. Psychological theory proposes that a new habit takes about thirty days to form, and my experience at Diet Designs bears this out. Unlike a quickie diet that encourages you to click out faster than you click in, the Portion Savvy 30-Day Plan is formulated to work with your cognitive structures to give you the healthy habits you need to become an expert food manager, eating just what you need to make your mind and body perfectly balanced and happy.

FROM COMMITMENT TO CONTROL

For many people, long-term conditioning and failed diets in the past combine to create a sense of learned helplessness. Bombarded with ridiculous quantities of food and the message that to eat it all is good, you naturally learn that food is less a matter of personal choice than it is an imperative, a force to submit to.

You are not helpless over your food choices. You are simply uneducated in the subject. Sure, you might know about the fat grams in butter, but few people actually know how much they need to eat to meet their energy requirements. This is what you'll learn with portion savvy.

The antidote to helplessness and hopelessness is gaining personal control, which is the goal of the Portion Savvy 30-Day Plan. You'll lose weight along the way, but even more important is what you'll gain: a new sense of mind-body control, based on proven behavior modification techniques, over your food.

Learned helplessness can be unlearned. Knowledge is power, and portion savvy is the force you need to manage food for life.

PART I

THE SCIENCE OF RIGHT-SIZE PORTIONS

THE PORTION PROBLEM

Denise came for her first Diet Designs consultation with thirty extra pounds of fat on her body but little extra fat to trim away from her diet. A busy executive in charge of foreign rights for a major movie studio, she made pasta with marinara sauce a mainstay of her business lunches, never touched chocolate, and even tried to work out as much as her schedule permitted. Sure, she had some soft spots and slipups in her eating regime, but in general, Denise was nutritionally aware and proactive in her habits. I could quickly tell that she'd walked into my office wondering what new trick I had to offer in her long-term battle with her weight. As a nutritionist in today's fad-driven diet environment, I'm used to that.

As always, I began by asking Denise to tell me what she ate on a typical day. And as usual, we never made it past breakfast.

"Cereal, nonfat milk, toast, and fruit." She looked victorious, sure that these healthy foods were above reproach. They *were* in the abstract, but it was the concrete details that mattered to me.

"Do you pour the cereal out of the box?"

"Well, yes." Denise stared at me as if I might be from another planet where cereal came in some other kind of container.

"Into any old bowl?"

"Into one of the bowls that I have," she pronounced carefully, as if to a small child.

"And the milk, do you pour it from the carton?"

"Yes . . . that would be correct." When I saw Denise looking at her watch and fidgeting, I knew I only had a minute to make it to the punch line.

"So how much cereal and milk do you think end up in your bowl?"

"What do you mean?" asked Denise, stumped and not liking it.

"In cups. How many cups of cereal and how many cups of milk?"

"I don't know . . . Maybe a couple of each? Less milk than cereal."

"Mm-hmm." I made a note. "And the toast?"

"No butter. Just marmalade!" she pronounced with a smile.

"How many slices?"

"Two."

My mental calculator was clicking. So far we were up to about 600 calories.

"And the fruit?"

She held out a fist, looked at it, then added the other. "Something between one and two of these."

That would tip the total up to about 750.

"And how many calories do you estimate your breakfast adds up to?"

Denise dealt in numbers every day and her answer was quick: "A few hundred."

"Try more than double that—and by my estimate, about half your daily allotment for maintenance of a fit body weight, without even getting into lunch and dinner. Even if your remaining meals are exactly aligned with your energy needs, you're putting on a pound a week from your extra breakfast calories alone."

I quickly jotted down the figures on a pad and showed her. The numbers spoke for themselves.

Denise, like so many before her, looked at me with both disappointment and relief. We were only at breakfast, and already the entire day was out of alignment. Like most people who care about their health and fitness, Denise was smart and attuned, and she knew: If the problem starts first thing in the morning, it's a big-picture thing. It needs a big-picture solution.

DENISE'S MORNING MISCOUNT

	Denise's Portions		Savvy Portions	
Cereal	2 cups	220 calories	1 cup	110 calories
Nonfat milk	1 cup	90 calories	$\frac{1}{2}$ cup	45 calories
Toast	2 slices	200 calories	$\frac{1}{2}$ English muffin	55 calories
Marmalade	2 tbsp.	90 calories	1 tsp.	15 calories
Fruit	$1\frac{1}{2}$ cups	150 calories	$\frac{3}{4}$ cup	75 calories
	TOTAL	**750 calories**		**300 calories**

$$750 - 300 = 450 \text{ extra calories/day} \times 7 \text{ days}$$
$$= 3{,}150 \text{ extra calories/week}$$
$$3{,}500 \text{ calories} = 1 \text{ extra pound of body fat/week}$$

Then we started to talk about miscounting calories. Denise was astonished to discover that she was typically taking in 800 calories at lunch, 1,000 at dinner, and 500 in snacks, adding up to a total of 3,050 calories per day. That was about 1,000 more than Denise needed to maintain her weight—let alone lose some, as she was trying to do through her low-fat diet. After a good hard look at the numbers, Denise's analytical mind led her to the inescapable conclusion:

"I've got a portion problem."

YOU ARE NOT ALONE

Nearly everybody miscounts calories. Clinical researchers who study food consumption patterns have found that Americans routinely underestimate their daily caloric intake by as much as 25 percent.[2] The most notorious underreporters are women and overweight people, suggesting a wishful-thinking component to this common behavior. Whether you run your daily numbers like a human calculator or just indulge in an occasional ballpark figure, chances are that you underestimate what you eat by up to 1,000 calories a day.

Food industry propaganda has eroded our portion sense with compelling catch phrases like "value meals," "all you can eat," "two for one," "jumbo," and "hearty." I recently bought a box of Cracker Jack at a Lakers basketball game and discovered that the one-ounce box of my youth has ballooned to eight ounces—meaning that my beloved and once-reasonable 110-calorie snack now costs me 880 calories! Restaurant portions are getting bigger every day, with many meals racking up 2,000 calories or more. To add to the problem, Americans are dining out more and more. The more you eat these supersize servings, the more you come to expect them at every meal.

Meanwhile, the federal government's Food Guide Pyramid is a well-intentioned attempt to improve the proportions of our diet, but its recommended numbers of servings from each food group have only compounded the portion problem. The Food Guide's servings are just a fraction of the real-life sizes found in packages, on store shelves, and on plates in restaurants. For instance, after stating that you should eat a generous-sounding six to eleven servings of grains per day, the Guide clarifies that a single bagel counts as two servings—and this is a two-ounce bagel, not the four- to five-ounce variety sold at most bakeries. In other words, eat a government-sanctioned bagel and you've had two servings of grains, but stop at one of the new bagel chains and you'll rack up five—and think you're eating only two. How is anyone supposed to know how much is enough?

It's the consumer who suffers in this behind-the-scenes battle over serving sizes. Einstein himself couldn't count correctly through all this conflicting information.

Evidence of the national miscount is all around us. One out of two Americans is now overweight, double the number of fifteen years ago. Three federal agencies—the National Center for Health Statistics at the Centers for Disease Control and Prevention, the National Institutes of Health, and the Department of Agriculture—track the food intake and body weight of Americans, and recent reports from all three groups indicate that we eat more and weigh more every year.

Even as the proportion of fat in our diet declines—dropping from 40 percent of daily calories in 1978 to 33 percent in 1996—the total number of daily calories that people eat continues to rise.[3] Food is energy, and the energy value of our daily diet jumped by 100 to 300 calories per day for various age and sex groups between 1980 and

THE PORTION PROBLEM IN PUBLIC

I recently did a survey of portion sizes at some of L.A.'s favorite restaurants to see how the false value of abundance was weighing down the plates. What I found were serious health violations invisible to the city inspectors:

➤ At a top steak house, the baked potato weighed in at twenty-two ounces, or nearly a pound and a half. That's 672 calories before you even dig into your T-bone! But take heart, spud lovers: *The portion savvy pop-outs will show you what a right-size potato looks like so you can trim it down to size.*

➤ At an elegant restaurant frequented by movie industry insiders, the swordfish steak weighed a full three-quarters of a pound, twice what anyone needs. *The pop-outs and the scale will help you get a handle on just how much fish will fulfill your personal energy equation.*

➤ The angel-hair pasta served at a well-known national restaurant chain totaled five cups, for an energy tab of 1,000 calories before adding sauce or Parmesan cheese. A national survey has found that the average restaurant portion of spaghetti with tomato sauce measures 3½ cups and costs you 849 calories. *Pasta is a notorious portion-problem food, and a simple measuring cup will help you master right-size pasta servings.*

1991. By 1991, the *average* intake for all Americans over two months of age clocked in at a whopping 2,095 calories![4] Current national calorie statistics are still being gathered and analyzed, but my experience at Diet Designs is that most clients are eating much more than that.

It's not that we're eating more in order to run more marathons. With 40 percent of Americans currently not exercising at all, we are as sedentary as seems possible. Our food needs are actually shrinking as our intake grows.

Body weight has inevitably followed the same ascending path as the calories in our diets. Between 1986 and 1993, the average twenty-something American adult gained ten pounds, creeping up from 161 to 171 on the scale.[5] At Diet Designs, I've found that people are just as likely to underestimate their weight as their caloric intake. Time after time, clients climb onto the scale for their initial weigh-in and exclaim, "What—I thought I weighed less!"

The reason for this widespread fattening-up is clear: Calories are energy to the body. Unused energy—*no matter whether it comes from fat, protein, or carbohydrates*—is stored as body fat. The extra 100 to 300 daily calories we accumulated between 1980 and 1991 could add a pound to your body as quickly as *every twelve days.* Add it up over eleven years, and we were lucky to get away with that ten-pound weight gain; theoretically, it could have been 330 pounds per person!

Fortunately, a number of other variables have intervened to prevent us all from weighing in at 400-plus pounds—but while there may be few other reasons to wish for a return to the seventies, I'd jump in a time machine if it could shave 300 calories off America's daily diet!

Our national obesity problem and its public health implications have become so dramatic that the federal government recently made headlines by issuing new, lower guidelines for healthy body weights. After decades of overindulgence, many Americans are shocked by the truth about what they should weigh for health and long life.

CALORIES COUNT MORE THAN FAT GRAMS

A Vanderbilt University study showed that calories count even when fat intake is limited. Two groups of overweight people were put on diets restricted to 25 grams of fat per day. One group ate as much as they wanted, while the other limited their calories to 1,200 per day for women, 1,500 for men. Five months later, the people practicing portion control had lost much more weight than those who didn't—18 versus 9 pounds for women, and 26 versus 18 pounds for men.[6]

Controlling calories can potentially *double* your weight loss over counting fat grams alone. That makes a good case for becoming portion savvy!

PORTION PERCEPTION

We're gaining weight as a nation because we're eating more energy than we expend. After more than a decade in nutritional practice and through dozens of diet fads, I've traced every client's problem, at base, back to portions. These are the phrases I hear:

➤ Late-night snacking.
➤ Afternoon depression.
➤ Sporadic schedules.

➤ Trigger foods.
➤ Feelings of fatigue.
➤ Fear of hunger striking before the next meal.

I've heard about every imaginable food-related dilemma from my clients. I listen, take notes—but mostly, I just wait, because I know that each client holds a secret inside. I wait for each one to make the most important discovery: Everyone, no matter what his or her emotional issues are, ends up telling me, "I guess I just eat too much."

It's a simple truth, but for many people, it's painful. Admitting that they eat more than they need not only feels like confessing a personal weakness, but also conjures up a grim vision of a future of deprivation and complicated calorie-counting that will never feel natural or fun.

My job is to educate my clients by explaining that their oversize eating blueprint is not a shameful flaw, but the result of very functional learning skills—and that those same learning abilities will help set them free from their battle with food. Once we've broken through the barrier of acknowledging the calorie miscount, the slate is cleared for a new picture, and at that point, here's what I tell my clients:

Most Americans are conditioned to overeat since birth.

From family patterns of presenting food as love, to those huge portions at restaurants, to the frenzied lifestyle that encourages a feast-or-famine attitude, our social and psychological surroundings have given us a mistaken message from the get-go: *More food is better, even beyond the point of physical satiation.* Well, more food is not better, and you can unlearn that message.

You're not weak or unintelligent for having learned this faulty lesson; in fact, your ability to learn and adapt has enabled you to learn this unhealthy habit. But the same skills you used to learn the wrong habits will help you learn the right ones. Applying your intelligence and your pattern recognition proficiency, which you use to establish repeated behaviors, you will become portion savvy.

Eating what's right for your body tastes and feels great.

If "going on a diet" has made you feel deprived in the past, prepare to reinvent your whole concept of what the word *diet* means. By matching your energy intake to your needs and giving you the tools to enjoy your favorite foods, portion savvy promises delicious meals, no hunger, and the natural vigor of good health. My clients repeatedly report that they feel the most satisfied—and the most vital and healthy—when they're eating Diet Designs food. When you get portion savvy, you'll have this experience every day.

"Thank God—portion control!" exclaimed my client Caroline when she came in to pick up her Diet Designs food after the Christmas holiday break. During those two holiday weeks without our quantity guidelines, her intake had gotten out of sync with her needs. She noticed that her energy and sense of well-being had suffered as a result. But even more telling, Caroline told me she'd had a hard time feeling *satisfied* from the large portions she ate during the holiday season. Not knowing her portion boundaries prevented her from deriving the pleasure she was accustomed to from Diet Designs meals. Constantly second-guessing whether she was eating too much and would regret it later, she couldn't have any fun with the flavors and sensations of her food.

For most of my clients, portion savvy is the ultimate safety net. It's the soft landing that leaves them free to enjoy food to its fullest. If you like to eat and want to be fit, full of energy, and around for the long haul, then portion savvy is your ticket to ride.

You don't have to count calories to control them.

Just as you don't notice the letters once you learn to read, becoming portion savvy will free you from the numbers in your personal energy equation. Once you've completed your training, you'll know how to identify your portions at a glance:

➤ A four-ounce piece of chicken.
➤ A plate of pasta sized to your stomach.
➤ The glass of juice that will give you a good dose of antioxidants without adding up to half a day's calories.

Once you accept that your instinct to eat has been inflated by a lifetime of misfired messages, you can get smart. You can get portion savvy. You will take your oversize eating blueprint and replace those erroneous images with the right ones. Soon you'll be remembering your personal serving sizes on automatic pilot. As you painlessly acquire new habits, you'll be moving toward your ideal weight, enjoying incredible energy, and eating delicious food without worries or guilt.

PORTION SAVVY: FAD-PROOF

Fad diets sweep the nation regularly and swiftly, and they seem to come even faster and more furiously in Los Angeles, where my practice serves some of the most trend- and body-conscious people in the country. Not a week goes by that one of my clients doesn't ask me about the latest craze, wondering whether I might add the food combination or diet drug of the day to my program. I'm happy to say that as steadily as I decline to do so, my clients remain faithful and successful for years on end.

In a roller-coaster business, being portion savvy is an oasis of stability because *portion control never fails*. Whether you ask satisfied dieters or a broad array of health and nutrition experts, calorie management lies at the heart of every success story. This scientifically proven practice has the legs to keep you fit for a lifetime.

Overeating has become a national health crisis and probably a personal crisis for you too. Portion savvy is a reeducation program to realign your mind and body with your diet and unlearn a lifetime of mistruths. I know that you can learn portion savvy because my clients do it all the time, painlessly and with lasting success.

My message as you ready your body and mind for an exciting new learning experience is a resounding "Yes!" You can—and you will—turn your portion problem into a new sense of *portion perception* that will bring you lifelong fitness and health.

CHAPTER 2

CALORIES COUNT

A calorie is a unit of heat used to express the energy value of food. When the number of calories you ingest as food and drink exceeds your daily energy requirements, the excess calories are stored as fat in your adipose tissue.

Simple, isn't it?

This basic equation explains why eating too many calories makes you gain body fat. What it doesn't fully describe are all the other ways that too many calories can make you sick and shorten your life—and how fewer units of food energy can promise better health and greater longevity.

Calories count because the number you ask your body to process every day has a direct impact on everything from body fat to blood sugar levels to the incidence of cancer. Research scientists have documented that when it comes to food-energy intake, less is definitely more. After decades of complicated diets and many more to come, you may be astonished at the evidence that the secret of a longer, leaner, and healthier life is as simple as whittling your daily calories down to size.

WHAT'S IN A CALORIE?

One calorie is the amount of heat required to increase the temperature of one kilogram of water by one degree Celsius. This is an absolute and unwavering measurement of the energy value of food—and whether it's from cucumber or bacon, a calorie is a calorie is a calorie.

To measure the caloric value of food in the lab, scientists use a device called a bomb calorimeter, an insulated chamber filled with oxygen and surrounded by a water bath in which they set food on fire and then measure the increase in the water's temperature. The heat released by the oxidation of food is known as the heat of combustion.

In the bomb calorimeter, the burning of one gram of pure carbohydrate raises the temperature of one kilogram of water by 4.2 degrees Celsius. Therefore, it contains 4.2 calories. The heat of combustion of a gram of protein is 5.65 degrees, and a gram of fat tops the charts at 9.45 degrees. Fat has a higher heat of combustion than protein or carbohydrate because it contains many more atoms of hydrogen than oxygen, which leaves the hydrogen free to oxidize and produce energy. (With me?)

For carbohydrate and fat, the heat of combustion of a particular food in the bomb calorimeter is equivalent to the energy released into your body when you eat it. A gram of protein, however, loses about a calorie when the body discards the unusable nitrogen in its molecules, leaving 4.35 calories available to the body, almost the same as for the carbohydrate gram. For simplicity's sake in nutritional calculations, these numbers are generally rounded off to four calories per gram for carbohydrate and protein, and nine calories per gram for fat. (Still with me?)

Because most foods contain a combination of carbohydrate, protein, and fat, their gram-for-gram calorie content varies with the mix.[7] Common portions for various foods are based on the caloric value of the nutrient mix they contain. The ultimate caloric yield of the nutrients in food is determined by the efficiency with which they are available to the body through digestion and absorption. That's the basic math you need to know.

CALORIES BY THE GRAM

The energy released into the body by food varies with its molecular makeup. Here are the calorie counts for the three different energy-producing constituents of food.

One Gram	Calories
Carbohydrate	4.20
Protein	4.35
Fat	9.45

SCIENCE SAYS LESS IS MORE

The only way to lose body fat is to eat fewer calories than you expend. For most readers, this is probably reason enough to cut back on their caloric intake. But there's more: Evidence suggests that eating less does your body favors beyond just letting you slip into a smaller dress or suit.

Reducing your caloric intake:

➤ Causes you to burn body fat and subsequently reduces your risk of serious diseases associated with being overweight, including heart disease, stroke, cancer, hypertension, and diabetes.

➤ Improves glycemic (blood sugar) control and increases insulin efficiency, helping to stabilize energy levels, nourish cells, and prevent the health risks of high blood sugar levels.

➤ Lowers levels of blood lipids (LDL cholesterol and triglycerides), which are direct risk factors for heart disease.

➤ Improves immune response, helping you ward off diseases from the common cold to cancer.

➤ Could increase good HDL cholesterol, reduce the age-related loss of DHEA hormone, and lower subcutaneous body temperature to slow aging and add years to your life.[8]

The pioneer studies on calorie restriction were conducted in the 1930s by Dr. Clyde McKay of Cornell University. Dramatically disproving the notion that animals naturally eat what they need, Dr.

McKay divided two groups of rats between a calorie-controlled regime and an all-you-can-eat smorgasbord. The animals given free rein gorged themselves—and died young as a result. The portion-controlled rats, however, lived longer and experienced lower incidences of cancer and vascular and kidney disease.

It's amazing, in retrospect, that evidence showing that eating less prolongs life has been around for more than half a century, and yet we're still trying to figure out what to do about it. The rest of this book will provide my specific recommendations on the topic, but first, let's consider the conceptual implications of McKay's work:

➤ McKay's fat rats tragically demonstrated that Mother Nature has not built a control mechanism into all her animals to prevent them from eating too much.

➤ Give rats more food than they need and they'll chomp it right down.

➤ In fact, confronted with an environment of abundance, rats eat themselves to death.

Is it any wonder, when huge portions of food are routinely crammed down our throats by everyone from clever marketers to our loving mothers, that humans do so too?

It's not that nature wishes ill health for rats *or* humans. It's just that our entire ecosystem is designed for species survival, not for individual longevity. No matter what kind of animal you are, the instinct to eat as much as you can allows you to grow, mature, and reproduce more quickly—which is great for the species, but lousy for your life span. You come and go quickly so that others may follow. Today, many individuals would probably agree that this live-fast, die-young schedule doesn't jibe with their hopes and dreams.

In the 1970s, Morris Ross of the Institute of Cancer Research in Philadelphia expanded on McKay's findings with further animal studies showing that calorie restriction improved immune response, reduced the incidence of heart disease and diabetes, stabilized blood sugar levels, and increased protein synthesis and turnover to better nourish cells and regenerate tissue.[9] Rats on restricted regimes lived 60 percent longer than those allowed to eat as much as they wanted.

CUT CALORIES TO LIVE LONGER: THE RESEARCH

➤ **1930s** Dr. Clyde McKay of Cornell University finds that rats given unlimited food will literally eat themselves to death, while animals on portion-controlled diets live longer with less disease.

➤ **1970s** "My rats are buff!" proclaims Morris Ross of the Institute of Cancer Research in Philadelphia. Dr. Ross's experiments find that rats on restricted diet regimes live 60 percent longer than those allowed to eat all they want and that they rate significantly better on a variety of health and longevity indicators.

➤ **1990s** Dr. Roy Walford tries calorie-cutting on people. Within six months of eating less in the Biosphere II, participants have lost an average of 22 pounds and cut cholesterol, blood pressure, blood sugar, and white blood cell counts. Further experiments with mice lead Walford to conclude that eating less could extend the human life span to up to 140 years.

➤ **2000 and beyond** Will you be one of the savvy eaters enjoying the antiaging benefits of eating for your energy requirements?

Furthermore, restricting food intake in adult rats was found to considerably overcome the risks of ad-lib feeding in early life, and the life-extending benefits of caloric restriction increased dramatically with age. The conclusion? It's never too late to start eating less.

Ross also found that cutting calories too much shortened his subjects' life span. This finding confirms the uncontroversial premise that eating too little leads to nutritional deficiency and impaired health. I'll talk more about the dangers of undereating later in this book, but I want to take this early opportunity to state that I do *not* advocate severe calorie restriction under any (nonclinical) circumstances.

Depriving your body of vital nutrients and energy is *not* portion savvy.

While Ross's discovery about the harmful effects of eating too little was unsurprising, there was an interesting wrinkle: The animals' health suffered even more when drastic restriction was imposed immediately after a period of overfeeding. In other words, rats are as adversely affected by crash diets as we are. These findings prove what a bad idea it is to overeat in anticipation of "going on a diet" or to attempt dramatic overnight changes in your eating habits.

In the 1990s, Dr. Roy Walford of the University of California, Los Angeles, took these decades of animal findings on the benefits of limiting energy intake and tested them on people.[10] His research site was the famous Biosphere II experiment, a three-acre, dome-enclosed, self-sufficient environment located near Tucson, Arizona. Biosphere was designed by a team of scientists to investigate many aspects of our ecosystem and our relationship with it—and Dr. Walford's particular interest was how restricting calories could affect human health.

From 1991 to 1993, Dr. Walford placed the eight participants in Biosphere II on a whole-foods diet that began at 1,800 calories and gradually increased to 2,200 calories per day. While these allotments are generous compared to portion savvy numbers, the Biosphere participants did heavy daily manual labor that increased their energy requirements significantly over those of most Americans. The men of Biosphere lost an average of 33 pounds on this regime to reach a body fat level of 6–10 percent, while the women slimmed down by a proportionate 17 pounds, with body fat averaging a lean 10–15 percent. Happily, the residents of Biosphere reported no undue hunger on their low-calorie diet—but the changes in their biochemistry were quite significant.

Though they were already above average in fitness levels when they entered the dome, the Biosphereans soon registered notable health benefits from eating controlled amounts of nutritious foods and leading a high-activity lifestyle: lower serum cholesterol, diastolic and systolic blood pressure, blood sugar, and white blood cell counts. Each of these indices is a direct risk factor in serious disease, and the team shaved off significant numbers simply by eating less and exercising more.

Like most studies, Biosphere II had some limitations and biases. The number of subjects was small and included the experimenter himself. The diet the Biosphereans ate was much healthier than the average American's, suggesting that some of its health benefits might have accrued from the selection of foods as well as their limited caloric value. The experiment has not been repeated or followed up. We haven't yet observed the effect of caloric restriction on humans

LOW CALORIE AND LOVING IT: BIOSPHERE STATS

Average Of	Before	After 6 months in Biosphere
Body Weight	148	126
Serum Cholesterol	191	119
Blood Pressure	109/77	76/57
Blood Sugar	92	70
White Blood Cell Count	6,600	5,000

over an entire life span—but Walford's work suggests that the results could be exciting when we do!

In addition to the Biosphere experiment, Walford has also conducted extensive animal studies on the effects of lower energy intake. He's found that mice who eat a calorie-restricted diet experience dramatically lower rates of breast, lung, and liver cancer, as well as leukemia. They also maintain bone mass longer and hold on to their youthful good looks, inasmuch as you appreciate the mouse aesthetic (healthy fur without gray, straight spines, and good grooming habits). They run mazes as fast as nonrestricted mice one-third their age and continue to make love and reproduce long after the rest.

Walford contends that controlling energy intake also boosts immune response, from liver and kidney functions to hormonal levels; protects your eyesight; and extends your athletic ability into your upper years. In short, he believes that eating moderately can cause you to age up to half as fast, and he postulates a life span of 120–140 years for people who do so—longer than the 110-year cap humans have historically confronted.

It's of paramount importance to note that while Walford's experiments cut calories, they also maximized nutrients, particularly vitamins and phytochemicals, minerals, fiber, protein, and omega-3 fatty acids. Biosphere residents ate vegetables, fruit, grains, legumes, meat, and fish. There wasn't a packaged or processed food to be found in the dome. As a result of this nutritious regime—Walford calls it the "nutrient-rich calorie"—the participants reported satisfaction even at calorie levels lower and activity levels higher than in life outside.

THE CANCER CONNECTION

Cutting calories could be a lifesaving defense against breast cancer. A study of mice with genetic markers for breast cancer found that a 40 percent calorie restriction significantly extended life span and inhibited the development of mammary tumors. Three years after the experiment began, nearly half the mice in the restricted group were still alive after all their free-eating comrades had died. Furthermore, tumor incidence was just 27 percent of the group, probably due to the higher expression of a tumor-suppressing gene and free-radical-scavenging enzymes observed in the low-cal mice.[11]

Other experiments with the effect of diet on mammary tumors in rats have found that *caloric restriction is even more important than cutting fat* to inhibit tumor development.[12]

In humans, a Harvard study has found that women who gained more than 45 pounds since age 18 nearly doubled their risk of breast cancer compared to those who had kept their adult weight gain within 5 pounds. Gaining 22 to 44 pounds increased the risk by 60 percent.[13] Researchers propose that the increased risk comes from high levels of estrogen, which feeds breast tumors—and which is produced by body fat. While this study addressed fat on the body rather than calories in, the only way to gain body fat is by eating more calories than you need.

I get the same sort of reactions at Diet Designs. My clients report with amazement how satisfied they are while eating delicious, nutrient-dense foods in smaller quantities than they're accustomed to. Many new clients can't believe that they're actually allowed to eat everything I give them, and they call me to second-guess the meal plan.

As you'll learn in this book, part of being portion savvy is choosing the foods your body needs and enjoying the satisfaction they naturally bring. Identifying the "nutrient-rich calorie" will soon become second nature—even as you learn to cut the occasional sliver of chocolate cake to nourish yourself in other ways.

Recently, further animal studies have affirmed that the health and longevity benefits of restricting calories extend to monkeys, providing good reason to believe that they translate to humans.[14] In sum, over half a century's worth of evidence gathered through the work of McKay, Ross, Walford, and other scientists suggests that eating less increases your resistance to disease and lengthens your life. Research has also suggested that while our eating instincts are regrettably programmed toward excess to sabotage our individual health and longevity, people can also be completely satisfied with a high-quality, low-calorie diet that delivers untold riches in fitness, vitality—life itself. Armed with this information, what are you going to do? Will you acknowledge that calories count . . . and make them count in your favor?

DROP POUNDS—AND PRESSURE

Could cutting calories also cut your need for expensive medications? Yes, if you're overweight and have high blood pressure. Many studies confirm that even small weight losses can lead to significant reductions in blood pressure in hypertensive patients—often enough to get off antihypertensive drugs, which carry risks and side effects of their own.[15] One of the most recent experiments, the Trial of Nonpharmacological Interventions in the Elderly, proved for the first time that the weight-loss/lower-blood-pressure connection holds true for older adults—and that a weight loss of as little as eight pounds can be enough to make these patients drug-free.[16] Since 60 percent of the population has high blood pressure by age sixty, portion savvy gets more important with each passing year!

Now that you know the many ways in which calories count, you'll probably be relieved to learn that *being portion savvy doesn't mean you have to add them up every time you open your mouth.* In fact, the whole purpose of getting portion savvy is to learn your serving sizes so that you can relax and enjoy your food while extending your life, enhancing your energy, contributing to optimal cellular and biochemical function, and freeing yourself from the heavy toll of overload. Once you understand and accept how calories count, you can move past calculating them to becoming right-size in your body and mind.

The National Weight Control Registry, a data bank run by Dr. Rena Wing of the University of Pittsburgh and Dr. James Hill of the University of Colorado, collects statistics from people who have lost at least thirty pounds and kept it off for at least one year. Participants in the NWCR report eating an average of just 1,380 calories per day, far lower than the national norm. These topflight food managers understand portion savvy, and about half of them say that maintaining their weight is actually easier than losing it was. This flies in the face of the usual diet statistics—and clearly demonstrates the huge chasm between following a fad diet, which is like cramming for an exam, and truly knowing the material.

You're ready now to understand your personal energy equation.

CHAPTER 3

YOUR PERSONAL ENERGY EQUATION

This is the math-and-science chapter. Don't skip it, even if you've always been math-and-science phobic. Understanding your personal energy equation is the first step toward being portion savvy for life.

Eating is energy to your body. Every bite of food you swallow supplies fuel to your cells, powering everything from your muscles to your brain, as gas does a car or electricity a lightbulb. Energy makes your body work and the world go around—but taking in more than you need can damage the very body you're trying to nourish. The first thing you need to do to get set for the Portion Savvy 30-Day Plan is to assess your personal energy needs. This chapter will tell you how.

Your daily caloric needs are determined by your personal energy equation: how many calories you typically expend, and whether you're trying to maintain equilibrium or burn fat for weight loss. Think of your body as the operational sign between the two sides of this equation. When energy in *equals* energy out, the equation is balanced and there's no change in body weight. When energy in *is less than* energy out, you draw upon stored body fat to compensate for the difference and lose weight as a result. And when energy in *is greater than* energy out, you store the extra as fat in your adipose tissue.

THE ENERGY BALANCE

Energy in < energy out: burn fat.

Energy in > energy out: store fat.

Energy in = energy out: no change in weight.

When you eat fewer calories than you burn through basic metabolic functions, daily activity, and exercise, your body draws upon the fat in adipose tissue for energy. Each time you run a caloric deficit, your cells turn to the fat you stored yesterday or last month or during your freshman year in college. When that happens, you lose body fat—and when the heat of combustion of fat burned totals 3,500 calories, you have lost a pound. That's what it takes: a deficit of 3,500 calories.

Every movement and internal process of your body is fueled by the energy contained in the chemical bonds in the carbohydrates, proteins, and fats in the food you eat. Your body's job is to liberate this energy by breaking the bonds, which it does with a series of chemical reactions in the mitochondria, or the energy centers of human cells. These reactions produce heat and a compound called adenosine triphosphate (ATP), the chemical currency that stores energy and powers bodily functions from blinking and breathing to running a marathon.

A burned calorie supplies heat and energy to your body. An unburned calorie turns to fat in your adipose tissue. Eat fewer calories than you expend, and you'll literally burn up that fat, providing all the heat and energy you need while making you more fit.

During the weight-loss phase of the Portion Savvy 30-Day Plan, you'll learn how to ensure that your energy input is less than your energy output for safe and efficient fat-burning. When you've achieved your goal, you'll move the equation into balance for lifelong equilibrium.

ENERGY OUT

As the energy equation demonstrates, the amount of energy you burn determines how much food you should eat every day, so I start all my clients with an overview of the output side of their personal energy equation. The variables in this number include your basal metabolic rate (BMR), how much you exercise, the thermic effect of the food you eat, and a process called facultative thermogenesis.

Basal metabolic rate.   Let's begin with the basics: How many calories does it cost you just to be you?

Your *basal metabolic rate* is a measurement of the energy expended for maintenance of normal body functions and homeostasis. The variables in your BMR include body size; body composition, or the proportion of lean body mass to fat; nutritional state; thyroid function; and sympathetic nervous system activity. In general, bigger (taller and/or heavier) people need more energy to run their bodies than small ones, and BMR increases with the proportion of muscle mass to body fat.

As the variables suggest, BMR can differ significantly with gender, age, and from one person to another. Your BMR accounts for 60–75 percent of your daily energy expenditure.

The number of calories required for the basic functions included in your BMR shrinks as you lose weight. As the output side of the equation decreases, so must your energy intake. But when you carefully calibrate your calories to meet your evolving needs, and when you protect and build lean body mass through exercise, you can counter the natural decline in BMR caused by weight loss. The Portion Savvy 30-Day Plan will teach you how.

Exercise.   One element of your energy output is completely under your control: exercise.

Simply speaking, exercise has been conclusively proven to be crucial to weight loss and absolutely indispensable to maintenance. Your activities—from scrubbing the floor to sweating at the gym—account for 15–30 percent of your daily calorie expenditure. Exercise burns fat in the present and keeps it off in the long term. Exercise is also strongly associated with the prevention of most life-threatening diseases, and it strengthens daily immunity. People who exercise are less likely to be overweight than those who don't, and regular activity

THE METABOLIC TRAP

The metabolism is programmed to maintain the status quo in the body. That means that when you run a calorie deficit, your metabolism does its best to spare calories. It simply asks your body to get by with less. Ever obliging, the body does.

Unfortunately, this mechanism is exaggerated by weight loss. A Rockefeller University study of men and women who had lost from 15 to 64 pounds found that they had to eat 220 to 300 fewer calories a day to maintain their new weight than people who had always been at that weight.[17]

The hard truth is that your body is going to resist your efforts to change it—*unless* you let your metabolism know who's boss. You do that by sticking to your interval eating schedule and getting plenty of exercise. The Portion Savvy 30-Day Plan has been specially formulated to get you past your natural metabolic hurdles, so follow the energy-burning instructions and feel those mitochondria at work!

appears particularly important in preventing age-related weight gain. The way exercise *rearranges* your body fat might be as important as its assistance in burning it: The improved waist-to-hip ratio that results from regular activity is linked with a lower risk of heart disease, hypertension, and diabetes. Even if you remain overweight, active people who carry extra pounds have lower mortality rates than sedentary overweight people do.[18]

Most experts recommend burning a minimum of 1,000 calories per week through exercise to support successful weight loss. That amounts to approximately two hours of jogging or three and a half hours of walking for most people, although individual rates differ. With over half the adult American population reporting that they exercise sporadically or not at all, this activity level is an excellent start.

But evidence suggests that this number is still on the low side for lifetime fitness. At the National Weight Control Registry, participants expend an average of 2,800 calories each week through exercise, which is equivalent to walking 28 miles. They also report that they started their exercise plan slowly as they first began to lose weight, then ratcheted up its intensity as they got more and more fit.

Exercise is an integral part of the Diet Designs program. Some of my clients, especially the busiest ones, protest. But when I show them the many studies proving how pivotal regular activity is to getting and keeping weight off; when I explain how just a little effort pays off in faster fat-burning, carefree maintenance, more energy, and a longer life to enjoy it in; and when I break the good news that exercise can actually make you *less hungry,* most agree to give it a try. Just like the converts at the NWCR, soon they're hooked and moving more every day.

This widely shared tendency to embrace an increasingly active lifestyle as you become more fit proves a basic portion savvy doctrine: *Big changes come from small changes.* Start slowly. When you give your mind and body time to accept and establish new habits, including exercise, positive behavioral results will follow.

The Portion Savvy 30-Day Plan will teach you how to manage the output side of your energy equation. You'll start slowly, conditioning your body to appreciate the joys of doing what it was born to do, then gradually and easily amp up the duration and intensity to arrive at an optimal level for fitness and motivation.

The exercise program in the Portion Savvy 30-Day Plan will help you to:

➤ Burn fat and lose weight more quickly.
➤ Feel more energized and less stressed.
➤ Break through hard times as you realign your habits.
➤ Build your resistance to minor illness and life-threatening disease.
➤ *Keep the weight off for life.*

One caveat: In case you should think you can dance off all your extra pounds without attending to your diet, it's been found that calorie restriction is still more important to weight loss than exercise. But the exercise edge remains all-important; in addition to helping peel off pounds faster than diet alone, a workout program enables you to burn body fat and spare your valuable lean body mass. Do your dieting on the couch alone, and you're as likely to lose muscle as your love handles.

THE EXERCISE POLICE

A study of the Boston Police Department put the officers on a diet, one group with exercise and one without. All the cops lost weight—an average of 23–27 pounds—but a year and a half later, the nonexercisers had regained more than 90 percent of the weight they'd lost, while the exercisers on average kept off *every single pound.*[19]

Food's thermic burn. Eating actually stimulates your metabolism!—not enough to compensate for the calories you take in, of course, or we'd all starve to death, but the metabolic boost you get from the *thermic effect of food* burns extra calories after every meal. When you eat at evenly spaced intervals, the thermic effect of food accounts for a sizable 5–10 percent of your daily energy output. The Diet Designs program has always included three meals and at least two snacks with strict instructions not to skip any of them. My clients are happily amazed by the satisfaction this timetable supplies and can't believe they're burning *more* fat while feeling *less* hunger than ever before. Interval eating is also one of the top strategies for the National Weight Control Registry members, who report eating almost five times per day.

EAT MORE OFTEN, BURN MORE CALORIES

Why settle for just two periods of thermogenesis, as do the many people who skip breakfast and eat just lunch and dinner, when you could fire up your inner furnace *five times* by eating three meals and two snacks per day? By maximizing the time your metabolism works at peak performance, you burn more calories, and hence more fat. Need I say more?

When you're running a calorie deficit, you need both the thermic boost and the blood sugar stability that interval eating offers. Many dieters make the mistake of spacing out their meals too widely, which can slow your metabolism, send your blood sugar below normal levels, and drive you to overeat at your next meal. The Portion Savvy 30-Day Plan will teach you to avoid this trap and take advantage of the fat-burning power of dietary thermogenesis with frequent, evenly spaced meals.

MAINTAINING THE FLAME

Like all metabolic functions, food's thermic effect changes as you age, and it looks as if as the years go by, you can only keep up your youthful postmeal burn by cutting the size of your meals and eating more frequently. A Tufts University study compared the metabolic impact of eating in two groups of women, one in their twenties and another that was postmenopausal (age fifty-plus). While both groups burned fat, protein, and carbohydrate at the same rate after meals of 250 and 500 calories, when the subjects indulged in 1,000 calories at once, the older women burned 30 percent less of the fat calories than the younger women did—just 187 versus 246. That 59-calorie differential could add up to six extra pounds of body fat each year.

  Older women can skip the annual six-pound weight gain and continue to burn bright by dividing their daily intake among more frequent meals of 500 calories or less.[20]

Facultative thermogenesis.   Have you ever wondered why you tend to get hungrier in the wintertime? It's facultative thermogenesis at work. Your metabolic response to ambient temperature and stress accounts for about 5–10 percent of your daily energy expenditure. Cold temperatures stimulate your adipose tissue to produce more heat to keep you from freezing to death—and in the process, you burn calories.

The extra energy demands of emotional stress also fall under this category. While stress is not a recommended weight loss method, facultative thermogenesis at least partly explains why high-stress moments lead to the munchies. You'll learn how to control stress-related eating in the Portion Savvy 30-Day Plan and protect the calorie-burning edge this thermogenic effect provides.

ENERGY IN

Once we've reviewed the output side of the energy equation, the burning question on all my clients' lips is "So how much should *I eat?*" Controlling the number of calories you consume every day lies at the heart of the portion savvy concept. But with every body being different, the number that makes your equation work varies from someone else's.

BOTH SIDES NOW: THE ENERGY EQUATION

The daily energy equation for a moderately active 5'4" woman weighing 150 pounds looks something like this:

Energy Input	Energy Output	
<2,000 calories = weight loss	Basal metabolic rate (75%)	1,503 calories
>2,000 calories = weight gain	Exercise (15%)	297 calories
2,000 calories = maintenance	Thermic effect of food (5%)	100 calories
	Facultative thermogenesis (5%)	100 calories
	TOTAL:	**2,000 calories**

Through the years of my practice, I've identified three different calorie levels that promote safe and effective weight loss without hunger or deprivation. I call these energy intake levels Portion Savvy 1, 2, and 3:

➤ PS 1 (1,200 calories per day) trims the fat off smaller body types, including most women, and people with slow metabolisms or sedentary lifestyles.
➤ PS 2 (1,600 calories per day) is the magic number for most men and some active or larger women.
➤ PS 3 (2,000 calories per day) ensures satisfaction and a safe fat-burning rate for people with very active lifestyles or more weight to lose.

I can't overemphasize the importance of matching your intake to your energy needs for efficient fat-burning. When your daily calories dip too low, not only do you run health risks ranging from nutrient deprivation to starvation, but you can actually shut down your metabolism so that it stops burning fat.[21] This same "fat-sparing" mechanism can also be activated by overexercising. That's why I've carefully formulated the PS levels and the workout program to meet all your nutritional needs while keeping your metabolism working at optimal efficiency.

I've also developed the Portion Savvy 30-Day Plan to deliver the right blend of nutrients for efficient fat-burning, healthy energy, and satisfaction. While calories are calories, balancing the nutrients in them is crucial to your health, performance, and long-term success.

The size of each meal you eat matters too. Taking in too much at once elevates blood glucose levels and makes digestion difficult. You'll learn the art of calibrating the flow of energy in with the Portion Savvy 30-Day Plan.

The most accurate way to match your Portion Savvy level to your body's energy needs is by measuring your basal metabolic rate. You don't need to go to a lab or get hooked up to a machine to find out how many calories your body burns for basic metabolic functions. You can approximate your BMR to within 10 percent of a laboratory measure with the easy calculation below.

Calculate Your BMR

1. Locate your height and weight on Scales I and II in the surface area graph on page 31. Use a ruler or straight edge to draw a straight line between the two points. Read the number where your line crosses Scale III. This is your body's *surface area* in square meters.
2. Identify the *hourly calories burned per square meter* for your age and gender:

	Women	Men
Age 20–40	36	38
Age 40+	34	36

3. Your BMR is your body's surface area multiplied by your hourly calories burned per square meter times 24 hours. Fill in your results from steps 1–3 in the equation below:

Surface area   _____
× hourly calories burned per meter   × _____
× 24   ×   24
= Your BMR   = _____

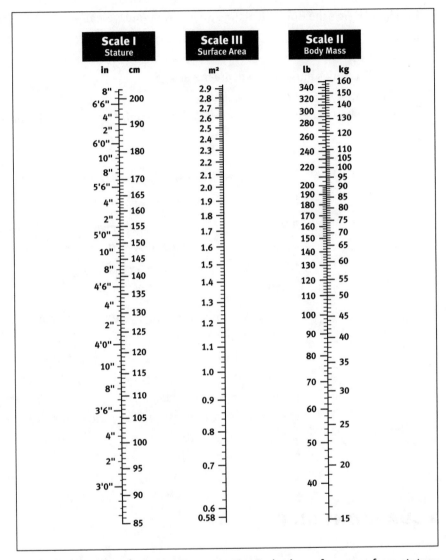

Surface Area Graph. Nomogram to estimate body surface area from stature and mass. (Reproduced from "Clinical Spirometry," as prepared by Boothby and Sandiford of the Mayo Clinic, through the courtesy of Warren E. Collins, Inc., Braintree, MA.)

Example: Here's the BMR calculation for a 35-year-old woman who's 5′4″ tall and weighs 150 pounds:

Surface area = 1.74
Hourly calories burned per square meter = 36
BMR = 1.74 × 36 × 24 = 1,503 calories
This woman's body burns 1,503 calories to maintain basic metabolic functions for a 24-hour period.

Now, use your BMR to locate your Portion Savvy level in the chart below.

BMR	Portion Savvy Level	Calories per Day for Weight Loss
<1,600	Portion Savvy 1 (PS 1)	1,200
1,600–2,000	Portion Savvy 2 (PS 2)	1,600
>2,000	Portion Savvy 3 (PS 3)	2,000

The woman in the above example would find herself in PS 1, eating 1,200 calories per day for safe, efficient weight loss.

By eating within your PS level and following the exercise program outlined in the Portion Savvy 30-Day Plan, *you should expect to lose eight pounds or more during the month you spend mastering portion savvy.* After that month, you've established the habits you need to continue losing weight until you reach your right size (more on that below) and then to maintain it for life!

YOUR RIGHT SIZE

Most Americans are in a double bind: We weigh more than we should, and yet we *think* we should weigh even *less* than we should. You can't win this way!

The first thing I tell my clients is to forget the idea that there's a magic weight that's going to change their lives, transform their body into Pamela Lee's or Jean-Claude Van Damme's or anybody's other than their own. There's no weight that will feel so instantly natural that it will maintain itself without effort. The best advice I can offer as a party to many weight-loss success stories is to turn your attention away from the number on the scale and turn it toward how you feel and look.

You'll try several self-assessment methods in the Portion Savvy 30-Day Plan, from the clothes-fit test to the naked-reflection-in-the-mirror test, all of which are powerful tools to help you decide when you've reached the right size. I've discovered time and time again that a healthy, sustainable weight must be *experienced.* Simply naming in advance a number that you're determined to achieve is counterproductive. Setting goals is important, but specific numbers are arbitrary and discouraging. Portion savvy is a process, and I encourage you to evaluate your fitness goal on an ongoing basis.

The variables in your right size include visible ones like gender and age—men generally weigh more than women because they're taller, have bigger bones, and carry more muscle mass; older people may find it increasingly difficult to maintain their youthful weight as their BMR declines with age. But there are less obvious factors too. Naturally muscular people weigh in heavier due to their high proportion of lean body mass. Genetics can influence each individual's propensity to store fat. Lifestyle and medical conditions can affect what weight is most realistic and healthful to maintain.

The simplest way to get a quick glimpse of your weight loss goal is to calculate your Body Mass Index (BMI), a number that relates your height and weight to assess approximately how much fat you carry. Something like a home version of a body fat test, your BMI allows you to relate your size to your fitness level.

To calculate your BMI, multiply your weight by 703 and divide the result by your height in inches squared.

Your weight $\times 703$ _____

$\div$ (Your height in inches)^2 _____

$=$ Your BMI   _____

Your BMI enables you to gauge how healthy your body weight is. Here are the ranges:

	Lean	Fit	Overweight	Obese
BMI	<19	19–24	25–29	30 and above

The goal of any weight loss program for health and well-being should be to attain a "Fit" BMI of 19 to 24, where your risks of developing diseases associated with excess body fat are significantly reduced.

However, within the wide range of BMIs considered to be fit, there are considerably increased health risks as you move toward the upper end. For instance, men with BMIs of 23–25 are at twice the risk for hypertension as those at 22 or less, while women at a BMI of 24 are five times more likely to develop diabetes than those at 21. In fact, diabetes for women is the disease most strongly associated with increasing BMI, and the steep curve doesn't level off until you get down to 21. For health and longevity, I recommend targeting a goal toward the bottom of the fit BMI range—but it's equally important to be realistic.

Here are some questions to add a reality check to the numbers on the chart.

➤ What weight have you maintained the longest after age 18?
➤ How long has it been since then?
➤ How do your lifestyle and goals today compare to that period?
➤ What clothing size would you like to be? One size equates to about 8–10 pounds.

I recommend that you identify a weight *range* as your goal. The Portion Savvy 30-Day Plan will walk you through ongoing self-assessments that help you gradually zero in on your right size. For now, follow the plan for your PS level, and your body will naturally move toward balance.

YOUR ENERGY EQUATION OVER TIME

The output side of your energy equation—the calories you need—can change with a variety of factors,[22] including:

➤ **Activity level.** Start biking to work fifteen minutes each way (200 calories total) and you can have an extra cup of pasta a day, or keep your servings the same and lose a pound every three and a half weeks. On the other hand, cancel your twice-weekly tennis date and you'll need to trim 68 calories (2 ounces of chicken breast) from your diet every day.

➤ **Weight loss.** Since losing weight cuts back both the rate at which you burn energy and the minimum amount required to make your body work, your leaner self requires fewer calories. To maintain efficient fat-burning as you lose weight, refer to the BMR calculation and PS level chart on pages 30 and 32. If you cross from one level to another, it's time to change your portion sizes! Spend at least a week retraining in the servings for your new PS level, and congratulations!

➤ **Age.** Again, metabolism works against you here, shaving your energy needs as the years advance, *unless* you compensate with enough weight-bearing exercise to maintain muscle mass. Generally, men's tendency to be overweight peaks between the ages of 45 and 54, while women as a group are increasingly overweight until they hit the 65-to-74-year-old range. Dr. Morris Ross found in his animal studies that the caloric intake most conducive to lengthening life span changed with age, with the benefits of restriction actually increasing from one age period to the next.

➤ **Pregnancy and nursing.** You definitely need extra energy to start a new life and feed a hungry baby! But this is no time to lose your portion savvy, since babies with fit mothers are healthier and have significantly less risk of being overweight themselves.

➤ **Illness.** Being sick generally reduces your activity and so trims back your energy needs. But good nutrition is never more important than when you're trying to heal! The nutrients in healthy foods boost immunity and promote tissue regeneration, so this is the time to make those nutrient-rich calories count.

To stay portion savvy through all your life phases, reassess your BMR and PS level with any of the above events. Your portion skills will last a lifetime; only the details will change.

THE MIDDLE-AGE MELTDOWN

Perhaps you've passed a certain age. Maybe you're thoroughly enjoying your prime and happy not to be a teenager anymore. But you may also have been mystified and none too pleased to notice that while your eating habits haven't changed much over the years, your body has—for the bigger.

Human metabolism naturally slows with age, and for many people the most noticeable change comes in middle age, when extra pounds seem to appear out of thin air. This metabolic slowdown is mostly attributable to a loss of muscle mass, which is a result both of age and of the decreasing activity typical of this life phase. Your body burns fewer calories to maintain fat than muscle—so let the biceps shrink and so do your daily food needs. That's how the pounds mount up.

Because men begin with more muscle mass than women, they suffer more from this age-related reduction in BMR. The daily minimum energy requirement for a 5'6", 140-pound woman drops only 40 calories from age 18 to 45 (from 1,510 to 1,470 per day), but a 6', 180-pound man sees a 145-calorie drop-off over the same time (from 1,939 calories needed per day at 18 to 1,794 at 45).[23]

The middle-age meltdown cries out for portion savvy! Now is the time to reassess your BMR and PS level, learn new portion sizes, and get back on the exercise bandwagon. Follow the Portion Savvy 30-Day Plan so you can enjoy your peak years with a spring in your step.

LONG-TERM MANAGEMENT

When you're portion savvy, there's no philosophical difference between losing weight and keeping it off. Once you get in the habit of choosing the foods and portions that work for you, fitness becomes a basic instinct. While the trick to losing body fat is unbalancing your personal energy equation, maintenance is all about beautiful, symmetrical balance.

To move from fat-burning mode to long-term management, simply switch from your last PS level for weight loss to the next one above (from PS 1 to PS 2, or from PS 2 to PS 3). Devote at least a week to consciously learning your new portions, then sit back and relax for a lifetime of health and vitality.

Getting to know your personal energy equation enables you to nourish yourself and enjoy your food without overdosing or going hungry. Energy is the force of life, and when you balance energy in with energy out, you have a healthy relationship between mind, body, and food.

CLICK IN

Your head might be spinning with energy-equation numbers right now, but the beauty of becoming portion savvy is that you'll learn to translate your energy needs into food on the plate without juggling a lot of figures. By focusing on portions, you can savor the *sensual* aspects of food and let the math take care of itself. It's easy . . . once you click in.

BEAUTIFUL BOUNDARIES

Audrey had a serious weight problem that went all the way back to her childhood. On the day of her first consultation with me she weighed in at 350 pounds and had been to every diet guru in town. Most recently, she had been derailed by a nutritional counselor who recommended "intuitive eating."

"You don't tell someone with an eating problem to eat whatever you want!" boomed Audrey. A top Hollywood agent, she had strong opinions and no patience for nonsense. "I need boundaries! I had no boundaries as a child!"

Audrey had lost both her parents when she was young, and without adequate guidance from her foster parents, she had simply followed her natural instincts and eaten as much as she could get her hands on. Audrey's story struck a nerve for me. The absence of my working mother from my own childhood had caused me to confront the same scary lack of limits, and my response to chaos in my early eating life had been to become a nutritionist. When I told Audrey this, we both ended up in tears. The lack of boundaries can hurt, and I've made my career out of setting limits that heal.

"I need rules, but I also don't need to be told that I'm bad when I break them," sighed Audrey.

I told Audrey that there were no good or bad foods and no eating behavior could make her a bad person. The boundaries set by portion savvy principles are designed to help make good health easy, not to punish. Part of becoming portion savvy is knowing that it's a process.

The Miller sisters were also in search of healthy limits. Never before had a trio of sisters come into Diet Designs and announced their united intention to follow my program to the tee. The three Millers were all attractive, professional women in their thirties, all recently broken up with boyfriends, all about twenty pounds over-weight, all really ready to make a positive and permanent change for themselves—and not one of them would know a right-size portion if it hit her over the head.

"Our parents worked," explained the sisters. "We had to fend for ourselves, and we were clueless. We still are and it shows. Can you help?"

All these women shared a strong craving: to know how much is enough.

"We're really committed—but we're a little too busy to do a lot of food math," said the Millers.

I reassured the sisters that controlling calories didn't mean counting them. And I told them all that I would help them find their healthy boundaries—simply by clicking in.

INTELLIGENCE: BETTER THAN INSTINCT

Humans are set apart from other species by our ability to improve upon instinct with intelligence. Instinct tells us the world is flat, but knowledge has found it to be round. It's an instinctual drive to mate with whoever's at hand when you're in heat, but humans have used their intelligence to identify the health risks posed by sex with random partners, and to value the personal, social, and spiritual benefits of committed, monogamous relationships.

Instinct may also drive us to overeat. From McKay's studies of rats back in the 1930s to contemporary experiments with people in all-you-can-eat situations, evidence shows that when faced with an abundance of food, humans and other animals regularly and predictably eat far more than they need. That old evolutionary mandate to live fast and die young is always trying to upset your energy equation with excess food. That's why you need to set your instincts aside and click in to your natural human ability to *learn*.

Clicking in means training your mind and body to identify your right-size servings—effortlessly, and with the confidence that comes of true knowledge. When you're learning to read, you click in at the moment in which letters become words, words become sentences, and sentences acquire meaning. When you're learning portion savvy, you click in when you *see* and *understand* what size your food should be. When your mind understands your energy requirements and makes choices in accord with them, your body becomes the healthy equals sign in the energy equation.

One of my clients described clicking in simply and best:

"I was looking at the chicken breast in my Diet Designs dinner," said Mark. "I'd seen a piece of chicken the same size in many other Diet Designs meals, under an assortment of sauces, with various things alongside, all tasting different, but all the same size. And all of a sudden, I went, 'Aha! So *that's* how much chicken I'm supposed to have!' "

From then on, Mark carried an image of that piece of chicken in his mind everywhere he went—to restaurants, while traveling, to meals at home and with friends. He never wondered or doubted again. In that instant, Mark had clicked in.

Learning portion savvy enables you to *assert your intelligence over your instinct:* Just as surely as you know that the world is round, you will eat in confidence that you're nourishing yourself for optimal health and longevity.

THE PORTION SAVVY MIND-SET

Clicking in *is* about knowing how much to eat, but it's *not* about counting the calories in your food. Counting calories doesn't work because studies show that most people count them wrong. And why wouldn't we? You can't see a calorie. You can't feel it or weigh it in your hand. While you might get some idea of a food's caloric density by its taste, there's no calculator on your tongue totaling up each bite you swallow.

So skip the complicated calculations and click in to your portion sizes instead. As you *move from miscounting calories to managing portions,* you'll find a new blueprint emerging in your mind, just like a photograph developing in the darkroom—a picture you carry with you everywhere to guide your eating choices.

As you measure portions in the Portion Savvy 30-Day Plan, you'll be surprised at how many different kinds of food end up fitting into one simple framework of serving sizes. Diet Designs has enabled me to boil the whole world of food down to a portioning science. Over years of controlling my clients' energy intake, I've come up with the right formula for sizing up chicken, fish, meat, pasta, casseroles, soups, stews, burgers, salads, side dishes, cereal, snacks, and desserts. Put them together in a well-balanced meal plan and voilà!—you're in your PS level.

At Diet Designs, I have a staff of ten serving over 150 clients twice a week. With fresh food that needs to be cooked, packed, and delivered within hours, the portioning system needs to be simple, replicable, and fast. Diet Designs runs smoothly as a production operation because portion savvy is practical . . . and the company enjoys success as a nutritional practice because portion savvy works.

PRESET PORTIONS: A DOUBLE BONUS

Studies show that it's natural to eat what's in front of you, regardless of your actual hunger and energy needs. That's why it's so important to decide how much you're going to eat *before* you sit down at the table. The premise is simple: Preset your portions and you can relax and enjoy your meal without second-guessing the state of your stomach or wondering whether another bite will blow your fat-burning efforts. It's completely safe. Effortless. Foolproof.

Many Americans suffer from our heritage of serving food "family style" from big communal dishes on the table that offer second helpings without even requiring you to move from your chair. While you might associate this serving style with pleasant images of shared abundance, let's face it: Few of us do the daily hard labor or face the threat of food shortages that created this custom. Portion savvy will teach you to plate your food in the kitchen, freeing you to have more fun with your family while you easily eat a meal that's just your size.

Another payoff of presetting your portions is that you can even savor some of the favorite foods you've been forgoing. The Portion Savvy 30-Day Plan will teach you how to grant yourself smart indulgences: a small portion of steak, a single scoop of ice cream, a special-occasion lobster with just a bit of butter. Controlled indulgences keep you on track, and when you're portion savvy, they're no problem.

MIND-BODY MEASUREMENT

Clicking in means turning abstract numbers into delicious food on a plate. As you follow the Portion Savvy 30-Day Plan, you'll learn first-hand how the servings that fit into your personal energy equation look, what they weigh on the scale or measure in a cup, which bowl in your cupboard holds your right-size serving of cereal, which glass is best for your juice, and why those big dinner plates might be sabotaging your best efforts.

The portion savvy click-in comes when your cognition and your senses, your mind and your body, work together to assess the food in front of you. As you practice and perfect portion savvy, you'll use four different types of mind-body measuring techniques that will make sizing up your servings automatic. These techniques include:

➤ **Visuals.**   Seeing is believing, and your eyes are a tool you carry with you everywhere. You've reached the highest level of portion savvy when you can visualize your servings. You don't have to budge your chicken breast from its plate or break out the measuring cups. Whether you use the portion savvy pop-out or the memory in your mind's eye, you see and you know.

➤ **Weight.**   The most exact and error-free way to measure food is by weight. Foods such as meat and seafood, dry pasta, cheese, baked goods, and many more don't lend themselves to measuring cups, but you can put anything on the scale. Because of its convenience and precision, weight is the standard measurement in professional kitchens, from Diet Designs to five-star restaurants. Many people are unaccustomed to using food scales at home, but once you get used to it, you'll wonder how you ever did without weighing.

➤ **Volume.**   Every cook relies on measuring cups and spoons for precise results from recipes, and now you'll learn how volume measurements can also offer precise portions for everything from yogurt and juice to cooked pasta, soups, stews, sauces, and side dishes.

➤ **Mind-body cues.**   Whether it passes through scales, cups, or tablespoons along the way, all the food in your diet eventually ends up in your body, which has its own ways of measuring what you've eaten. Cues such as stomach feel, energy, and mental alertness can tell you when you've reached your optimal energy intake. The catch is that it's too late to cut back oversize servings when your food is already swallowed—and to add insult to injury, *there's a fifteen-minute lag for your satiety signals to kick in.* Portion savvy will teach you how to preview your body cues and use them in tandem with other measurement techniques to reinforce how *right* right-size servings feel inside.

The tools you'll use to master the portion savvy measuring techniques include the unique visual pop-outs in this book, a kitchen scale, measuring cups and spoons, and your mind and body. You'll experiment with each on a variety of foods. You'll doubtless encounter some unexpected surprises. And soon, you'll click in.

Every healthy relationship has boundaries. Steady, stable, secure, life-affirming boundaries. The sort your mom set for you. The kind you establish with a mate to navigate sticky issues, and with your children to keep them safe and instill good values. The same types of routines and expectations you establish at work so that you can stay sane and do your best job. Your only hope for lifelong fitness is a healthy relationship with food—so by clicking in to portion savvy, you're going to bring boundaries to your plate.

Now let's get savvy.

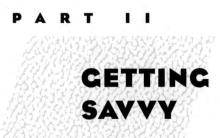

PART II

GETTING SAVVY

THE PORTION SAVVY 30-DAY PLAN

THE HEART OF A GOOD HABIT

The Portion Savvy 30-Day Plan is based on the proven framework of behavior modification. Many studies show that the key to long-term weight loss is a systematic program to change behavior.[24] Results for programs that couple behavior modification with healthy, calorie-controlled menus are significantly better than for diet alone; likewise, nutritional education alone has proven insufficient to make people lose weight, and diet drugs soon lose their effectiveness without a heavy-hitting behavioral plan.

In other words, people need to *do*. Clinical research and my experience have proven that to lose weight and keep it off, you need to take action, practice, experience firsthand, walk the walk, and self-talk the talk. Modify your behaviors and before you know it, you have an airtight habit that will have you thinking and doing the right thing for your fit self without missing a beat.

Behavior modification is the systematic manipulation of all the factors associated with your behavior patterns—in this case, those that pertain to eating and exercise. A good behavior-based diet addresses the personal, emotional, and motivational factors that contribute to eating behaviors and provides the tools to overcome obstacles on all these fronts.

The elements of eating behavior can be described as:

➤ Sensory-motor: your physical experience.
➤ Language-cognitive: what you think and how you process events, including self-talk.
➤ Emotional-motivational: how you feel.[25]

The Portion Savvy 30-Day Plan works on these three levels with explicit instructions on what to physically *do* along with the information that will help you *understand* and targeted input on how to manage the way you *feel*.

FIVE STEPS TO FOOD MANAGEMENT

There are five components to a behavior modification diet, all of which you'll encounter and implement in the 30-Day Plan:

1. **Self-monitoring.** By observing and recording the situational factors, thoughts, and feelings that surround your eating experience, you gain the self-knowledge you need for greater control. Many studies show that self-monitoring supports weight loss and maintenance.[26] With the Portion Savvy Plan, you'll keep a daily food journal that gives you this extra edge.

2. **Stimulus control.** Reducing the environmental cues that lead to overeating frees you from the external triggers that can take over your better judgment. The Portion Savvy Plan helps you clean up everything from your kitchen to your plate.

3. **Contingency management.** Otherwise known as rewards for good behavior, contingency management requires that you give yourself nonfood payoffs when you stick to your eating and exercise plan. Sorry—one of my strict rules is that you must enjoy yourself!

4. **Behavioral change.** This is the heart of the Portion Savvy Plan. You'll learn to consistently preset your portions to match your energy needs, choose the most satisfying and energizing foods, cut fat, and eat at regular intervals. You'll

repeat these behaviors every day. Soon, you'll have new habits.

5. **Cognitive self-acceptance.** The state of mind you bring to a problem directly influences your chance of overcoming it. You've got to feel good about yourself to believe that working for change is worthwhile. If there's one thing I've learned working with high achievers in Hollywood, it's that even the most seemingly confident people can keep up a steady stream of negative self-talk that limits their success. The Portion Savvy 30-Day Plan will help you rethink the idea that excess food is self-nurturing. You will reverse your old negative self-statements and come up with your own notion of safe and healthy boundaries.

WHY THIRTY DAYS?

Psychologists hold that thirty days is the time frame required to establish new habits. I follow this schedule at Diet Designs, where every new client receives four weekly consultations with me to lay the groundwork. I've found that for most people, a month of guidance is just right—not so much that it's intimidating to take on, yet enough to teach the necessary new skills and create a feeling of confidence and safety. It's the time it takes to wean off overeating and evolve toward energy balance.

Just about everyone can make a commitment for a month, and I've found that in those all-important thirty days, I can help people develop new relationships with food that last for life.

STAGES OF CHANGE

All learning requires change. As you follow the Portion Savvy 30-Day Plan, you will be changing your behaviors. I've asked for and have received that commitment from every one of my clients, and now I need to ask for it from you.

Change is a positive force. It allows you to reach your goals and realize your dreams. Change is a constant and inevitable fact of life. It can also conjure up fear and anxiety, and I've seen people get defensive at the very mention of the word.

I'm not asking you to change your *self*—just your habits and some negative thinking patterns. A habit is no more than something you do repetitively. It doesn't define you, and so setting out to change it needn't threaten your sense of who you are.

Your habits don't define your inner essence, but a good one, such as brushing your teeth, can make a critical difference in your life without requiring much conscious effort on your part. It's simple: You brush your teeth every day, your smile remains intact, and you have minimal encounters with the dentist's drill.

Of course, you might not remember, but it takes some doing to learn how to brush your teeth the first time around. So does portion savvy, which is a higher-level habit than keeping your teeth clean. Portion savvy is more like reading: It is based in knowledge and cognition as well as repeated behaviors. That's why I ask you to spend thirty days acquiring the habits and the understanding. I also ask you to take it slowly.

At Diet Designs, I've found that people who start too fast—people who are overzealous, obsessed, or trying to make too many major changes at once—tend to last about two weeks and then drop out. They never make it to the magic thirty days at which habits become ingrained. It's like trying to run before you can walk or to understand a sentence before you can sound out the words.

Likewise, psychologists speak of "stages of change," or the natural transitions that people tend to go through as they take on something new. Generally, you start with the status quo, then get to thinking about making a change. You go on to make definite plans to do so, and when you're ready, you start to actively modify your behaviors. Once you've tweaked and tuned everything to your liking, you move into the final stage of change: living and enjoying your new habits.

Researchers have found that for a weight loss program to succeed, the information and steps presented in the plan must correspond to your stage of change. Small, daily steps match the intensity of the strategy to your readiness to change, and both accelerate in tandem.[27]

My clients come to me at all different stages of readiness. Some have done their inner work and they take off running. Others ease into the program gradually, their enthusiasm growing as the results take them by surprise. Many new clients have sky-high expectations but haven't yet made a commitment to change. People who are fired by hope but not ready to actually do the work tend to be diet-hoppers, and I tell them that I intend to be their last stop.

I can make such a claim to everyone, regardless of readiness, because I've found that my program segues smoothly through all the stages of change and can engage you wherever you are. Howard is a case in point.

Howard came to me on a dare from his grandchildren. He told me he'd take off his extra weight to show them how much he loved them, but he had every intention of putting it back on later, and he told me so. "I love food," said Howard. "End of story. Now give me your diet."

Seventy-five pounds later, Howard had learned the unthinkable: He could eat less and be perfectly satisfied—happy even, and healthy and proud. Despite his promise to return to his old ways, Howard stuck with the new habits and kept his weight off. "Well, I guess I'd like to be around to see those grandkids grow up," he said.

Howard did the work, and the motivation followed. Some things in life just seem to run in reverse.

Changing your eating habits can be hard. If it weren't, we wouldn't have such a weight control problem in this country. But permanently transforming your eating habits and your body for the better is not only perfectly possible, it can actually be easy with the right tools and a program that encompasses the psychological and physiological facts of what it is to be human.

The Portion Savvy 30-Day Plan is designed to get you ready as you go—so no matter what stage of change you're in, you'll move on with increasing motivation and resolve.

A lot of the words that help you succeed in any learning situation start with *C*. I use some of these C-words to define the stages of change represented by the Portion Savvy 30-Day Plan. You'll take on one each week:

Week One (Breakfast):	**Commitment**
Week Two (Lunch):	**Challenge**
Week Three (Dinner):	**Concentration**
Week Four (Bringing It All Together):	**Control**
Graduation (Launch Your New Life):	**Calm**

Be patient with yourself during this gradual, step-by-step process. Small changes add up to big ones. You learned to walk one step at a time, and there was a lot of practicing to do before you started running. *Expect less and achieve more!*

PLAN MECHANICS

Here's an overview of what you'll be doing for the next thirty days:

➤ You'll tackle one meal per week—breakfast in Week One, lunch in Week Two, and dinner in Week Three. The fourth week will have you putting all three meals together, and you'll graduate from the program by learning to create your own meal plans.

➤ Each day tells you exactly what to eat for your portion savvy level, along with:

• Hands-On, specific portioning instructions that you can use as models for many different meals. The cross-sensory experience of weighing, seeing, and feeling food in your body internalizes the messages of each lesson.

• High-Nutrient Eating, a quick briefing on how the foods of the Portion Savvy Plan maximize your energy and extend your life.

• A Savvy Kitchen Strategy to keep your kitchen work under control.

- Tips and anecdotes that help you take your portion savvy skills to restaurants, treat yourself to special indulgences, and more.
- Portion Savvy Empowerment: motivational hints, behavioral strategies, affirmations, and other ways to encourage teamwork between your mind, body, and emotions for eating well.

➤ The behavior at the base of being portion savvy is *measuring,* whether with your eyes, a scale, or measuring cups. You'll use the following tools every day in the Hands-On segment of the Portion Savvy 30-Day Plan (I recommend purchasing any missing items before beginning the program):

- The portion savvy pop-outs in this book, unique visualization aids that enable you to quickly size up a chicken breast, a potato, and many other items on your meal plan.
- A kitchen scale.
- Measuring cups, dry and liquid.
- Measuring spoons.

I prefer a large kitchen scale with a knob you can turn to zero to adjust for the weight of a dish; a few sets of nesting, metal dry-measuring cups and spoons; and an assortment of clear-glass liquid-measuring cups that provide full visibility and can go into the microwave.

➤ The weekly workout: Each week features an exercise program designed to work with your meal plan to gradually increase the output side of your energy equation. You'll follow the natural stages of change with an easy start, then add intensity as your body becomes increasingly energized. By the end of the 30-Day Plan, you'll be exercising for optimal fat loss and long-term maintenance.

PORTION SAVVY FOOD

Each day, you'll eat three meals and two to four snacks, depending upon your PS level. Here's a reminder of how to find your PS level based on your BMR.

BMR	Portion Savvy Level	Calories per Day for Weight Loss
<1,600	Portion Savvy 1 (PS 1)	1,200
1,600–2,000	Portion Savvy 2 (PS 2)	1,600
>2,000	Portion Savvy 3 (PS 3)	2,000

Here's how the daily energy intake breaks down for each PS level:

Daily Calories by Meal and PS Level

	PS 1	PS 2	PS 3
Breakfast	300	350–400	450–500
Snack	—	100	100
Lunch	350	450	550
Snack	100	100	100
Snack	—	—	100
Dinner	350	450	550
Snack	100	100	100
TOTAL	**1,200**	**1,600**	**2,000**

No matter what your PS level, each day is carefully calibrated to provide the balance of nutrients you need for energy, cell repair, tissue building, immunity—all the good things that food does for you!

Daily Composition of the Portion Savvy Plan

Carbohydrates	Protein	Fat
60%	20%	20%

Each day of the Portion Savvy 30-Day Plan provides instructions for preparing and portioning a certain type of popular meal—pasta, meat and potatoes, sandwiches, lasagna, and everything else you love to eat. Some meals are quickly assembled from store-bought ingredients, others draw upon delicious Portion Savvy Recipes, and all can be varied to suit your tastes. There are vegetarian alternatives for those who prefer them. My bottom line is that food should be delicious and eating a joyous experience, and part of a truly balanced energy equation is satisfying your individual desires.

So enjoy the meals outlined in the Portion Savvy Plan, then simply add snacks according to the above schedule and the Portion Savvy Snack List on pages 210 and 211. Snacks keep your blood sugar stable and your metabolism going strong. They prevent you from feeling starved when you sit down to meals, which is a sure formula for overeating. The Portion Savvy Snacks are built into the daily energy intake for your PS level and they're fun! So whether you like savory or sweet tastes, crunchy or creamy textures, don't skip your between-meal pick-me-ups.

YOU'RE SET UP TO SUCCEED

Below are some characteristics of successful behavior modification programs and how the Portion Savvy Plan delivers them.

To change behavior you need:

- Well-defined target behaviors.

- Localized intervention in the spot where the behaviors take place.

- Tools to enable the target behaviors.

The Portion Savvy Plan provides:

- Daily, detailed portioning assignments.

- Practice in your own kitchen and dining room, at the office, and in restaurants.

- An assortment of mind-body measurement tools; nutritional lessons that provide proof of the importance of eating well; behavioral and cognitive techniques to support the click-in to a new mind-set.

THE 24-HOUR BALANCE

Your body has rhythms just like the sun and the moon, and when it comes to balancing your energy equation and meeting your nutritional needs, you have a 24-hour window to work with. From a physiological standpoint, the precise composition of each meal and snack is less important than your 24-hour tally of calories, vital nutrients, and energy expenditure. This isn't an excuse to skip meals all day and gorge at dinner, but it is a license to leave behind your worries about micromanaging, for instance, the protein-carbohydrate balance of a single snack. Don't sweat the small stuff: Just stick to a portion-controlled, interval-eating schedule, incorporate a variety of foods into your diet, and balance the energy book daily.

Ready for Week One: Breakfast—and commitment? Let's get started on your healthy new habits.

WEEK ONE: COMMITMENT

BREAKFAST

The first meal of the day can get you on the way to forming a whole new portion perception before you're even fully awake. This week, you'll focus on healthy, right-size breakfasts that fire up your metabolism for efficient fat-burning all day, provide the physical energy and mental alertness you need to take advantage of your peak morning hours, and offer a quick and easy wake-up to your taste buds. In starting your day right, you'll **commit** to becoming portion savvy so that each daily beginning can blossom into the lifelong healthy habits proven to realize your best potential.

While breakfast is the only meal you'll measure during this introductory week, I ask you to take some simple additional steps that will put weight loss immediately into gear. Portion your breakfasts and follow the guidelines below, and I promise you'll see the pounds start to melt away.

Week One Game Plan

➤ Portion your breakfast according to the following plan, and for the rest of the day, cut out as much as you can of the following:
  - Bread (except in sandwiches)
  - Desserts (except for designated Portion Savvy Snacks)

- Added fats—butter, mayonnaise, oil, and full-fat dairy products (milk, cheese, cream, sour cream, etc.) Substitute nonfat or low-fat dairy products, fat-free salad dressing and mayonnaise, mustard, salsa, Tabasco or Worcestershire sauce, lemon or lime juice, vinegar, herbs, and spices.

➤ Eat your designated number of snacks between meals (see the Portion Savvy Snack List on page 210), spacing them out for steady energy and metabolic burn.

Subsequent weeks of the 30-Day Plan will teach you how to incorporate everything you love into your diet. For now, just make these small adjustments, concentrate on your commitment to becoming portion savvy, ease into the exercise plan—and enjoy your first week of learning and losing!

PORTION SAVVY EMPOWERMENT

The portioning practices you'll learn in the coming weeks are the repetitive behaviors that will make balancing your energy equation an easy and healthy habit. Along the way, you'll engage in some additional activities and cognitive exercises that will take portion savvy beyond a measuring process and ingrain your new knowledge deeply into your consciousness. I call these practices Portion Savvy Empowerment—proven ways to build a fit mind-set and enhance your personal power over your energy balance.

You'll start with four empowerment activities that will extend throughout the 30-Day Plan. In addition, every day of the plan will offer a booster shot for your new mind-set. Armed with these high-impact learning techniques, you'll acquire portion savvy far more easily than you learned algebra. Getting and staying fit is not brain surgery!—but you do need the right tools.

Assess yourself.   The first part of making a commitment to change is taking a good look at where you are now. Take the following physical assessments to serve as a benchmark by which to measure your progress.

➤ Weigh yourself first thing in the morning, either without clothes or always wearing the same thing.

➤ To calculate your BMI, see the equation on page 33.

➤ To take your measurements, use a cloth measuring tape to measure the girth of each of the spots designated below. Use moderate tension on the tape and read the number where the lines cross. Don't hold your breath, flex your muscles, or pull the tape tight. Take your measurements once a month only, to give your body time to change.

➤ For the clothes-fit test, select some garments that fit snugly. Put them on and see how they feel. Use these same clothes for the fit test in coming weeks.

Weight_____   BMI_____

Measurements
Chest (at widest point)   _____
Bicep (at widest point)   _____
Waist ($\frac{1}{2}$" above belly button)   _____
Hips (stand with feet together and
    measure at widest point of buttocks)   _____
Right thigh (just below buttocks)   _____

Initial clothes fit test (fill in the size):
_____ Pants   _____ Skirt   _____ Shirt or blouse   _____ Blazer or jacket

Present weight goal range _____

Set goals.   One thing I know from my practice is that people's true motivation for losing weight runs much deeper than a dress size or a number on the scale. I ask you now to set some goals for undertaking the Portion Savvy Plan that reflect your most closely held life values.

Why do you want to become fit? To have more fun with your children? Put more energy into your job? Enjoy life on this planet for longer? To live in the image that your spiritual practice suggests?

Take a piece of paper and write down all your goals for becoming portion savvy, from large to small. Don't edit yourself—just brainstorm. You'll have a chance to rewrite your goals as you go.

Start a food journal.   One of the best-documented techniques for crafting better eating habits is keeping a food journal, in which you record everything you eat and any important thoughts, emotions, or circumstances that relate to your eating experience. This helps to hold you accountable to yourself in the present, to track patterns over time, and to provide a reliable record of your progress.

Designate a notebook or diary as your food journal. Date every day and make an entry after each meal and snack that notes what you ate and in what quantity. Then ask yourself:

➤ What was I thinking before, during, and after that meal?
➤ How was I feeling? Rate yourself 1–5 for depressed to happy, then repeat for tense to relaxed; write these ratings down and note any other emotions.
➤ What was going on in my day or in my life that affected my meal?
➤ What choices did I make that I feel good about?
➤ What regrets or concerns do I have about the meal?

Write down the answers to any of these questions that seem relevant. Don't worry about what you say or how; this is your private journal, a safe and privileged place where you can say anything you feel or think.

Your journal is also a great place to jot down the results of your weekly self-assessments, so that you can keep track of your progress all in one place.

Right now, fill the first page of your journal with the most meaningful goals from the list you just brainstormed.

Start a scrapbook.   Your portion savvy scrapbook is a visual record of thirty wonderfully important days in your life. Keeping your scrapbook will train your visual cognition and provide a reliable reference for the future. Here's what you do:

➤ Buy a scrapbook, some rubber cement, and a few rolls of film.

➤ Have someone take your snapshot today. This doesn't have to be a glamour portrait—just a candid photo of you right now.

➤ This week, take a picture of each of your portion savvy breakfasts after you have them portioned and served.

➤ Take another picture of yourself at the beginning of weeks 2, 3, 4, and 5.

➤ Photograph each meal you portion in upcoming weeks— lunch in week 2, dinner in week 3, and breakfast, lunch, and dinner in week 4.

➤ As you develop your film, paste the photos into your scrapbook with the date of each picture and any notes you want to make.

➤ Refer to your scrapbook anytime you forget what your right-size portions look like. Share your snapshots with friends and family so they can better understand your new habits and mind-set. Display your scrapbook as proud evidence of your accomplishment; treasure it as a memento of an important transformation in your life.

WORKOUT: WEEK ONE

This week, you'll leverage the value of your portioning lessons with an easy exercise program that burns calories and boosts metabolism for maximum fat-burning and a healthy heart, arteries, muscles, and bones.

Exercise is a great jump start to weight loss. In one of nature's few favors to people with pounds to lose, you actually burn more calories in any weight-bearing activity the higher your body weight is. For example, a 180-pound person expends about 534 calories in an hour of tennis, compared to 372 calories burned by a person who weighs in at 125.[28] So the light, weight-bearing workouts you'll enjoy during this first week pack an extra punch, pumping up the output side of your energy equation to eliminate pounds fast—especially if you plan your session for about half an hour after a meal or snack to take advantage of the added thermogenic, or calorie-burning, power of your meal.

Meanwhile, the portion savvy workout plan improves your health in other ways. Just walking at three miles per hour can raise your levels of "good" HDL cholesterol, and exercise has been shown to significantly reduce the amount that your triglycerides (blood lipids implicated in heart disease) rise after eating.[29]

Let the healing begin!

Portion Savvy Workout, Week One

Burn at least 200 calories on each of five days of this week with one or more of the following weight-bearing exercises:

Weight-Bearing Exercise	Calories Burned per Half Hour*
Walking (4 mph)	140
Treadmill or stair-stepper	200
Jogging	240
Low-impact aerobics	170
High-impact aerobics	240
Golf	150
Tennis	240
Soccer	240
Downhill skiing	170
Cross-country skiing	270
Ice or roller skating	240
Ping-Pong	140
Bowling	100
Frisbee	100
Yard work	170
Heavy household cleaning	150

* By a 150-pound person.[30]

MONDAY, DAY I: THE WELL-BOUNDED CEREAL BOWL

It's amazing how many of my clients get off on the wrong foot with the simple mistake of the bottomless cereal bowl. Here's how to start the day right-size with the classic quick breakfast of cereal, milk, and fresh fruit.

Breakfast, Day 1	PS 1	PS 2	PS 3
Fat-free or low-fat breakfast cereal	1 oz.	1½ oz.	2 oz.
Skim milk	¾ c.	¾ c.	1 c.
Fresh fruit	1 med.	1 med.	1 med.
Calories	**290**	**325**	**450**

Hands-On

➤ **1 medium fruit** =
½ banana, grape-
fruit, or mango
¼ papaya
15 grapes or cherries
½ cup berries

1. *Weigh the dry cereal into the bowl.* All cereals are not alike! While Total costs just 83 calories per cup, a denser cereal such as Grape-Nuts squeezes 400 calories into that same amount of space. But the scale is the great equalizer. Simply *put your bowl on top, turn the knob to zero, and add cereal to your allotted weight.*
2. Remove the bowl from the scale, *measure your milk into a liquid volume cup to the amount indicated for your PS level,* and pour it in.
3. *Place the portion savvy pop-out over your piece of fruit* to determine if it's "medium" size and trim it down until it fits. See the guidelines to the left for some special cases.

High-Nutrient Eating: Fabulous Fiber

Breakfast cereal is a good place to get high-quality fiber—both the soluble kind, which can lower your cholesterol and cancer risk as well as slow the release of glucose into the bloodstream, and insoluble

THE PORTION SAVVY POP-OUTS

The portion savvy pop-outs make sizing up your servings quick and easy. Whether you're portioning fruit, chicken or meat, fish, rice or grains, potatoes, or muffins, the pop-outs help you measure your right-size serving *and commit its image to memory*. Simply remove the pop-outs from the page along the perforations for your PS level and hold them over your food. If you see edges sticking out from underneath the pop-out, your portion is too big. Use a knife to trim away the edges until the shape of your portion matches the pop-out. You're training your eye while you trim off excess calories!

fiber, which stimulates your digestive system and provides an immediate sensation of fullness in the stomach. In fact, one experiment found that when people were given a breakfast of cereal and orange juice, those who had the highest-fiber cereal ate 150 calories less on average than the rest and took longer doing so.

The government recommends that you get at least 25 grams of dietary fiber each day, about double the average American intake. Start on your daily roughage requirement with cereals that provide at least 3–5 grams of fiber per serving, such as shredded wheat, Grape-Nuts, raisin bran, All-Bran, oatmeal, or Roman Meal apple-cinnamon.

IT'S IN THE BOWL

Find the bowl in your cupboard that most closely accommodates your portion of cereal—more likely a dessert than a soup bowl! Note the levels of your cereal and milk as you pour them in. By the end of the month, you should be able to skip the measuring cups and use your special bowl as your gauge.

Savvy Kitchen Strategy

Enjoy a quick, hot, one-bowl breakfast by cooking oatmeal or other hot cereal right in a (microwave-safe) bowl in the microwave. In general, a bowl of oatmeal will cook up in 1½–2 minutes on high, or see package directions.

If you like the instant oatmeal in individual packets, remember that each packet contains an ounce—which makes measuring for your PS level a snap.

Portion Savvy Empowerment: Natural Rewards

A basic premise of behavior modification is that rewards for good behavior reinforce those actions, encouraging you to repeat them until they become established habits. The most potent reward is a "natural" one, a simple activity or item that adds pleasure to your daily life.

➤ Sit down now and make a list of twenty small things, unrelated to food, that make you happy: a hot bath, a new magazine, calling an old friend, a movie or your favorite soap opera, a good book or listening to a symphony all the way through.
➤ For the next two weeks, reward yourself with one thing from your list for each day that you stick to your portion savvy eating and exercise plan.
➤ Don't skip your rewards! They're an important factor in establishing new habits—and you deserve them!

TUESDAY, DAY 2: TAMING THE MIGHTY BAGEL

One reason for the bagel's popularity is its prodigious size. Many bagels weigh in at four ounces or more—and while you might not dream of eating four slices of bread, it's no problem to munch down their caloric equivalent in one of these big guys, often spread with several portions of cream cheese. Today you'll learn how to tame the bagel with your kitchen scale to keep that fistful of bread from becoming fat on your body.

Breakfast, Day 2	PS 1	PS 2	PS 3
Bagel	1 oz.	2 oz.	2 oz.
Fat-free cream cheese			
OR Chive or Fruit Spread*	2 T.	3 T.	3 T.
Orange, grapefruit, or tomato juice	½ c.	¾ c.	1 c.
Nonfat milk (in cappuccino)	½ c.	½ c.	1 c.
Calories	**240**	**388**	**463**

* See the Portion Savvy Recipes beginning on page 157.

Hands-On

1. *Place your bagel on the scale.* If your bagel weighs more than your PS level calls for, cut it in half or scoop out the inside until you reach your target weight. Toast it if you like.
2. *Use a tablespoon to measure your cream cheese or spread,* leveling each spoonful off with a knife.
3. *Pour your juice into a liquid measuring cup,* then into a small juice glass.

JUST JUICE

Note the level of your juice in the glass, then use the same glass every time. By the end of the month, you should be able to gauge your juice without a measuring cup.

4. *Pour your milk into a liquid measuring cup,* then heat it in the microwave, on the stovetop, or with a cappuccino foamer, and mix with hot brewed coffee or espresso to taste.

High-Nutrient Eating: Fruit Juice

Your portion savvy serving of juice might be less than you're accustomed to drinking. That's because fruit juice packs a high caloric punch—but if you choose the right kind, it also jams in the vitamins. Skip grape and apple juice, which are high in sugar and low in nutrients, as well as cranberry, which contains added corn syrup or artificial sweetener. *Orange and grapefruit juice* are my best bets, both loaded with the antioxidant and immunity-boosting vitamin C. (Note that grapefruit juice can interact with certain medications; consult your prescription labels or pharmacist.) Orange juice is also rich in folate, an essential B vitamin that most Americans are short on, and is often fortified with calcium, which the vitamin C helps your body to absorb. The folate count of juice from frozen concentrate is just as high as from fresh, so you can take advantage of its convenience and economy at no nutritional cost.

Tomato juice is a good alternative if you like a savory taste in the morning, but be sure to buy the reduced-sodium kind. Absolutely avoid "juice drinks," which are mostly sugar and do nothing to launch your cells on an action-packed day.

THE WET AND THE DRY

Some recipes and portion savvy instructions distinguish between dry and liquid volume measurements. Though there's no difference in the actual volume involved—a cup is a cup (is eight liquid ounces)—dry measuring cups are designed to be filled to the top and leveled off, while liquid measuring cups mark graduated measurements up the side of the cup and usually have a lip at the top to help you handle liquids without spilling. They might give the fluid-ounce equivalent of cup measurements. Don't confuse liquid ounces with ounces of weight!

1 cup = 8 fluid ounces
3/4 cup = 6 fluid ounces
1/2 cup = 4 fluid ounces
1/4 cup = 2 fluid ounces

NO FREE SWEET NOTHINGS

Fruit and fruit juice are the healthiest way to indulge your sweet tooth. In addition to supplying important phytochemicals and fiber, fruit is naturally sweetened with fructose, the only simple sugar that's metabolized in the liver and so doesn't accumulate in such high concentrations in the bloodstream. This spares you the insulin highs and lows that table sugar (including brown and natural sugar), honey, molasses, and rice syrup can cause.

Once you separate fructose from the fruit, as in powdered fructose or the many "fruit-sweetened" products on the market, you lose fruit's nutritive value and are left with only empty calories. If you must sweeten your food, I recommend fructose over other forms of sugar because it's easier on your glycemic levels—but any form of sugar is a high-calorie food, and it will pack on the pounds if you overindulge.

I don't advocate trying to fool your sweet taste buds with artificial sweeteners. Some, such as saccharin, are known to pose health risks, while the long-term effects of others such as aspartame remain unknown. Furthermore, it's proven that artificial sweeteners fail to help people lose weight. Perhaps the biggest threat to your long-term health posed by fake sweeteners is their false message: that you can continue to feed your addiction to nonnutritive food at no cost to your well-being. The only surefire route to a long life of good health is to cultivate your appetite for healthy, nutrient-dense foods in portions sized to your energy needs.

Enjoy your delicious fruit juice and remember that there are no free sweets.

Savvy Kitchen Strategy

If you buy fresh bagels, weigh and cut or scoop them to your portion size when you get home, wrap well in plastic, and freeze. You can pop your right-size serving directly from the freezer into the toaster for many mornings to come.

CAFFEINE AND COFFEE DRINKS

Current evidence indicates that the caffeine present in one cup of coffee or tea a day doesn't present a health risk—but you *can* sabotage yourself by ordering supersized concoctions with added milk, sugar, or whipped cream. A large café mocha can have as many as 409 calories and 31 grams of fat—so while you may think you're just wiring up, you're actually drinking an entire breakfast's worth of calories. If you like cappuccino or latte, have a small with nonfat milk, and if it's not on your portion savvy menu, count it as a snack.

Portion Savvy Empowerment: Affirm Your Commitment

After your portion savvy breakfast, take a minute to say the following affirmation aloud:

By taking this first step, no matter how small, I'm on the right track to better health and well-being.

Write the affirmation on a small card and carry it with you today, stopping to reread it anytime you need a boost.

Try making a tape of yourself speaking your affirmation; pop it on while you drive or play it on your Walkman before a workout. Make yourself heard.

WEDNESDAY, DAY 3: BEATING EGGS' BAD RAP

Scrambled eggs are delicious, but the type served at a greasy-spoon diner will trip up your calorie control efforts with the day hardly begun. Here's a version you can enjoy for the rest of a long, healthy life.

Breakfast, Day 3	PS 1	PS 2	PS 3
Egg whites	4	6	8
OR nonfat egg substitute	¼ c.	6 T.	½ c.
Chopped vegetables	1 c.	1 c.	1 c.
Toast	1 slice	1 slice	2 slices
Pure fruit preserves	1 t.	1 t.	2 t.
Fresh fruit	1 med.	1 med.	1 med.
Calories	305	337	485

Hands-On

1. *Separate the prescribed number of eggs and discard the yolks,* reserving the whites, *or pour nonfat egg substitute into a liquid measuring cup.* With a fork, lightly beat eggs with salt and pepper to taste.

2. *Chop enough vegetables of your choice to fill a one-cup dry measure.*
3. Dab a little safflower or canola oil onto a paper towel and rub onto the bottom of a small nonstick skillet. Place the skillet over medium heat, add the chopped vegetables, and sauté until just tender-crisp. Turn heat to low, add the egg mixture, and scramble until set.
4. Meanwhile, toast the bread. *Measure the fruit preserves with a teaspoon* leveled off with a knife. *Size up your fruit with the portion savvy pop-out* or see the list of equivalents on page 63.

High-Nutrient Eating: Eggs

True to their bad press, whole eggs contain a concentration of saturated fat and cholesterol—but when you throw the yolks away, you've got a great start to a portion savvy day. Egg whites are unique in the world of food as a fat-free source of complete protein, which is what you need to build and repair cells and tissues, release alertness chemicals in the brain, and maintain your immunity. Most egg substitutes are egg whites with a few things added to mimic the missing yolks, so if you prefer their flavor, texture, or color and don't mind spending more money, go right ahead. Look for brands specifying natural preservatives and coloring agents.

Scrambled eggs also offer an excellent excuse to get some vegetables into your breakfast. It's never too early for the health benefits of veggies!

Savvy Kitchen Strategy: Separating Eggs

Separating egg whites from their yolks can require a few practice runs for the uninitiated: Crack the egg right across the middle with a sharp rap on the edge of a metal bowl. Hold the egg over the bowl and catch the yolk in one half of the shell, pulling the other half away and letting the white fall into the bowl. Tip the yolk back and forth from one shell half to the other until all of the white has separated itself, then throw the shell and yolk away. An alternative is to use an egg separator, available at kitchen stores.

Use the portion savvy paper towel trick described in step 3 of Hands-On to oil a nonstick skillet any time you sauté. It's almost fat-free and spares you the additives and fluorocarbons of cooking sprays.

Choose the vegetables for your scramble from what you've got on hand—onions, peppers, tomatoes, mushrooms, spinach, summer squash, broccoli, and so on. If you've got leftover steamed veggies from dinner last night, use them and skip the sauté.

MORNING MEAL REDUCES FAT'S APPEAL

A Michigan State University study found that women who ate breakfast were more likely to keep the day's fat consumption within 30 percent of calories than those who skipped—and in general, breakfast eaters have an easier time controlling their weight. Fuel your body when it needs it, and you can tame your fat tooth without even trying!

Portion Savvy Empowerment: Act As If

Your inner biorhythms and changing life circumstances combine to ensure that your energy for any project comes in waves. Just as you can enjoy riding the highs, you also have to wait out the low ebbs, trusting that your belief in your goal and your will to pursue it will soon return without any effort on your part.

During the first part of the Portion Savvy Plan, your primary job is to "act as if." Behave as if you're already portion savvy and in perfect control of your food. Your apparent obstacles will melt away, and your motivation will grow every day.

Persistence + faith = act as if

THURSDAY, DAY 4: THE MEGA-MUFFIN

Why is the muffin such a morning favorite? Because many muffins are more like a big slice of cake, with all the fat and empty calories, than they are a sensible breakfast. The portion savvy muffin is "mega" only in its nutritional profile and its power to energize your morning.

Breakfast, Day 4	PS 1	PS 2	PS 3
Low-fat, whole-grain muffin			
OR Cherry–Oat Bran Muffin*	1 (3 oz.)	1 (3 oz.)	1 (3 oz.)
Diced fresh fruit	½ c.	¾ c.	1 c.
Low-fat cottage cheese	⅛ c.	¼ c.	¾ c.
Calories	310	358	473

* See the Portion Savvy Recipes beginning on page 157.

Hands-On

➤ 2 tablespoons = ⅛ cup
4 tablespoons = ¼ cup
8 tablespoons = ½ cup
12 tablespoons = ¾ cup

1. *Place your muffin on the scale and trim it down until you reach your target weight.* Discard the excess. If you've followed the recipe in this book, your muffin should weigh in at three ounces—but check just to be sure.
2. *Dice enough fresh fruit to fill the dry measuring cup(s) appropriate to your PS level.*
3. *Measure your cottage cheese with a dry measure*—or if you prefer, use a tablespoon instead. Top the cottage cheese with the fruit.

High-Nutrient Eating: Beautiful Bran

Bran is one of the best parts of the grain, the place where most of the fiber and vitamins B and E are found—and yet most grain products you eat have had the bran stripped away. While this may create a softer, lighter (and more boring) product, you also miss out on wheat bran's ability to prevent colon cancer, diverticulosis, irritable bowel syndrome, and hemorrhoids, or oat bran's power to bind with fats in the blood and escort them out of the body.

Your breakfast muffin is an early opportunity to enjoy the nutty taste and chewy texture of bran, along with the tummy-filling fact that *wheat bran expands fifteen times in your stomach.* But beware. Just because a muffin is brown doesn't mean it contains bran. If you didn't make it yourself, read the ingredient list.

In fact, many commercial muffins are made mostly of sugar and contain little nutritive value. The healthiest muffin is packed with whole grains and fruit with little to no added fat.

Savvy Kitchen Strategy: Freezing and Reheating Muffins

Whether you've baked up a batch of muffins or brought home a box from the grocery store, it's smart to circumvent temptation by wrapping and freezing them right away. Wrap each muffin individually in plastic and freeze in resealable freezer bags. To serve, place the wrapped, frozen muffin in the microwave and cook on defrost for one minute, then on high for thirty seconds or until heated through. Unwrap carefully and let cool a few moments before eating.

MEMORIZE YOUR MUFFIN

If you prefer to pick up a muffin from your favorite bakery, coffee shop, or breakfast cart, use this portion savvy trick to tackle the potentially huge calorie count: Buy the muffin you like best (low-fat and whole grain, please!), bring it home, and place it on the scale. Cut it to your portion size, discard the extra, and stare hard at your trimmed-down muffin until the size is engraved in your mind. Take a knife to your office or wherever you eat breakfast, and from now on, cut your muffin to size from memory, immediately giving the extra away or crumbling it into the wastebasket.

Portion Savvy Empowerment: Enjoy

Today, take a moment to experience what a joy healthy eating can be. Sit down and eat your breakfast without the distraction of television or the newspaper. Enjoy and savor this ritual.

Take some time today to appreciate the support your family members can offer in your healthy eating efforts—and to recognize the challenges they can present. Food and family go together, and the optimal pairing of the two results in healthy meals shared in an atmosphere of love and fun. Let your family know how they can help you in your progress toward becoming portion savvy—and if they're getting in your way, gently ask them to step aside.

FRIDAY, DAY 5: YOGURT AND FRUIT

Do you ever wake up craving something sweet and creamy? This breakfast will make your dreams come true, and you could almost do it with your eyes closed.

Breakfast, Day 5	PS 1	PS 2	PS 3
Sweetened, nonfat yogurt	1 c.	1 c.	1 c.
Diced fresh fruit	½ c.	¾ c.	1 c.
Low-fat cereal (granola, Grape-Nuts, etc.)	½ oz.	1 oz.	1½ oz.
Calories	300	375	450

Hands-On

1. *Open an 8-ounce carton of yogurt OR spoon yogurt into a one-cup dry measure.*
2. *Dice enough fresh fruit to fill the appropriate dry measuring cup(s) for your PS level.* Combine the yogurt and fruit in a bowl.
3. *Place your bowl on the scale and turn the knob to zero.* Slowly sprinkle in cereal up to your allotted weight.

High-Nutrient Eating: Get Milk!

Calcium is a miracle mineral. Not only does it build and maintain strong bones, thereby reducing the risk of being crippled by osteoporosis, but calcium has also been found to lower blood pressure. In fact, a recent study revealed that a diet rich in plant foods and low-fat dairy products can lower blood pressure as much as antihypertensive medication does, and the calcium-rich diet was nearly twice as effective as a vegan diet in bringing blood pressure down.[31] Researchers believe that calcium might lower blood pressure by helping the kidneys release sodium and water.

Unfortunately, most Americans don't get enough calcium from their diets, and the absorption rate from supplements averages only about 60 percent. That's why you need to get milk—or yogurt, cheese, or buttermilk, the richest sources of calcium—every day. Dairy products are a good food once you take out the fat, and the Portion Savvy Plan gives you a daily dose in the morning.

Include some strawberries or oranges in this morning's fruit mix and their vitamin C will help you absorb more of the yogurt's calcium.

YOGURT: THE REAL DEAL

Yogurt makes a convenient and nutritionally winning breakfast or snack when you choose brands that are real food rather than sugary desserts. Here's what to look for:

➤ Nonfat. Full-fat and even low-fat yogurt can be as rich as sour cream.

➤ Live and active cultures, which help digest the lactose in milk and add helpful bacteria to the alimentary tract. This criterion knocks pudding-style "yogurts" such as Snackwell's out of the running.

➤ No add-ins other than fruit. Eating yogurt doesn't constitute an excuse for adding candy or cookies to your breakfast.

➤ Fruit juice or fructose sweetener. While to your body, sugar is sugar, fructose hits your bloodstream a little slower than table sugar, so go with fruit-sweetened if you're subject to sugar highs.

Portion Savvy Empowerment: Visualize Success

Success comes more easily when you see it. It's time to picture your portion savvy self.

Sit down, close your eyes, and breathe deeply for a few minutes until you feel relaxed. Now, visualize these scenarios:

➤ You, ten (or twenty or thirty) pounds lighter. How do you look? How do you feel? What are you wearing? How do you move? How do the people around you behave? How do you interact with them? As this scene unfolds, allow it to reveal any fears you might hold about being thin. Now, gently guide your visualization to see yourself as loved, confident, happy, healthy, energized, and fulfilled.

➤ Imagine you a month from now—if you should choose *not* to become portion savvy. You're eating without a plan and outside of your energy equation. How do you look and feel? How do you behave with other people?

Use your mind's eye to focus your energy on health and well-being, and what you see will become what you are.

SATURDAY, DAY 6: GREAT SHAKES

Wake up with a shake! Fresh fruit and soy are a fast way to stoke up on supernutrients—and if you're in a real rush, you can even sip your breakfast while you drive.

Breakfast, Day 6	PS 1	PS 2	PS 3
Light vanilla soy beverage	1 c.	1½ c.	2 c.
Protein powder	2 T.	2 T.	2 T.
Fresh fruit	¾ c.	1 c.	1¼ c.
Calories	295	380	465

Hands-On

1. *Pour the soy beverage into a liquid measure,* then into the blender.
2. *Measure the protein powder with a tablespoon* and level with a knife. Add to the blender.
3. *Roughly chop enough fresh fruit to fill the dry measuring cup(s) for your PS level.* Add to the blender along with ice to taste and whir until thick and creamy.

High-Nutrient Eating: Superfood Soy

There ought to be a law that everyone eat soy. Not only does it give you essential nutrients such as calcium, iron, zinc, phosphorus, magnesium, vitamin B_{12}, niacin, folacin, and the only complete protein in the plant world, but soy can also save your life. The phytoestrogens (plant versions of the hormone) in soybeans appear to block breast, ovarian, and endometrial cancers as well as keep calcium in your bones and alleviate the symptoms of menopause. The compound genistein found in soy also seems to cut off cancerous tumor growth. And studies suggest that soy foods can lower your cholesterol, which in turn cuts your risk of heart disease. In sum, soy is on the must-eat list for both men and women.

Unfortunately, most of us are unaccustomed to the joys of soy and have a hard time incorporating it into our daily diets. That's where a great shake made from soy beverage and isolated soy protein powder can help. Quick and delicious and good for everything from your blood to your bones, a soy shake is a smart start.

Savvy Kitchen Strategy: Freezing Fruit; Favorite Soy Picks

Frozen fruit makes a shake whip up frosty and thick—so today, why not take your leftover chopped fruit, portion it, wrap it in plastic, and pop it in the freezer for next time? This works especially well with bananas and solves the problem of what to do with the extras. Frozen fruit also makes a good snack all by itself.

When you're shopping for soy beverage, I recommend Westsoy Vanilla Light (or your favorite brand at about 120 calories and 2.5 grams of fat per cup). Look for a protein powder made from isolated soy protein, containing about 100 calories and 24 grams of protein in a two-tablespoon serving; I like Naturade Vanilla.

BEWARE OF THE JUICE BAR!

Juice bars are sprouting up like superpollinated weeds, and though they might appear to be healthy places to grab a quick energizer, portion savvy people approach the juice bar with extreme caution. The first thing they notice are the gargantuan size of the servings, many times your morning juice portion and easily adding up to hundreds of calories in juice alone. Then there are all the fattening add-ins: frozen yogurt, syrups, and powders that make these drinks more like milk shakes (and meals) than juice (or a snack). And the menu of nutritional supplements purported to have magical tonic properties? Most of them are patently unproven, probably a waste of money, and in some cases perhaps even a risk to your health.

If you like to get your breakfast shake at a juice bar, find one that offers a small size of 8–12 ounces or split the shake with a friend. Skip the add-ins and stick to fresh fruit, soy beverage, and protein powder. And remember: This is a meal!

Portion Savvy Empowerment: Clean Up the Environment

You've probably heard of the see-food/eat-food diet. The plan is simple (and not recommended): Eat everything you see. Our natural tendency to let environmental cues shape our eating behavior is actually based in the body; exposure to the sight and smell of food has been found to change people's insulin levels, which can in turn predispose you to overeat.[32]

To prevent this uninvited attack on your hormonal balance, today's the day to make your eating environment clean and healthy by clearing out the cupboards, refrigerator, freezer, and any hidden stash spots. Take out all your "trigger foods": unhealthy items filled with fat, hydrogenated oils, calories, or sodium such as chips, pretzels, cookies, and candy. These are often supplies you tell yourself you need to have on hand for unexpected guests. Throw these triggers away.

CHICKEN
BREAST

FRUIT

GRAIN/PASTA
SIDE DISH

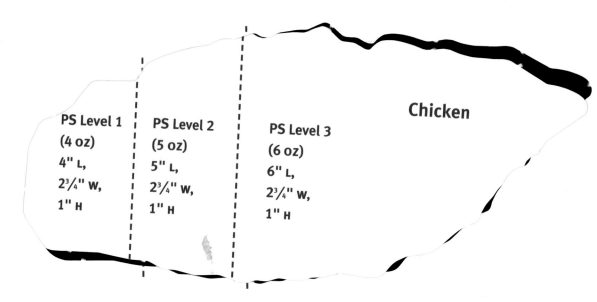

PS Level 1
(4 oz)
4" L,
2³/₄" W,
1" H

PS Level 2
(5 oz)
5" L,
2³/₄" W,
1" H

PS Level 3
(6 oz)
6" L,
2³/₄" W,
1" H

Chicken

Grain/
pasta side dish

PS Level 1
(½ C) 3¹/₄" DIAMETER, 1¹/₄" H

PS Level 2
(³/₄ C) 3¹/₄" DIAMETER, 1³/₄" H

PS Level 3
(³/₄ C) 3¹/₄" DIAMETER, 1³/₄" H

Fruit
PS Level 1, 2, 3
(Med) 3" W, 3" H

Muffin

PS Level 1, 2, 3

(3 oz) $3\frac{1}{4}$" DIAMETER, $2\frac{1}{4}$" H

Potato half

PS Level 1, 2, 3

(4 oz) 4" L, 2" W, $1\frac{1}{2}$" H

Fish

PS Level 1: (5 oz) 6" L, $1\frac{1}{2}$" W, 1" H

PS Level 2: (6 oz) 6" L, $1\frac{3}{4}$" W, 1" H

PS Level 3: (8 oz) 6" L, $2\frac{1}{4}$" W, 1" H

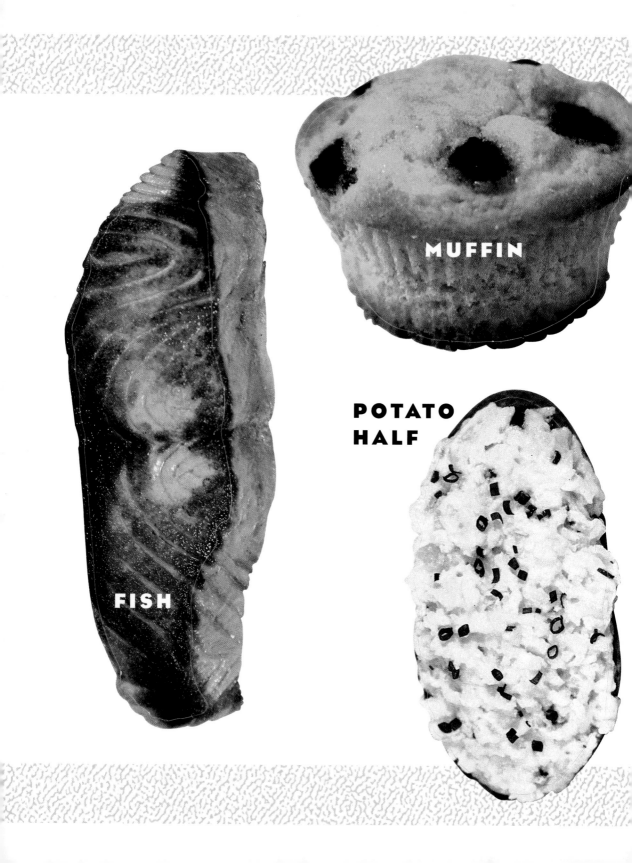

MUFFIN

POTATO
HALF

FISH

SUNDAY, DAY 7: GET YOUR GRAINS

A cross between the comfort of hot cereal and the decadence of dessert, Multi-Grain Pie is a power breakfast you can make and portion in advance.

Breakfast, Day 7	PS 1	PS 2	PS 3
Multi-Grain Pie*	1 piece	1 piece	1½ pieces
Orange, grapefruit, or tomato juice	½ c.	¾ c.	1 c.
Nonfat milk	1 c.	1 c.	1 c.
Calories	**261**	**336**	**444**

* See the Portion Savvy Recipes beginning on page 157.

Hands-On

1. *Cut the Multi-Grain Pie into nine pieces* by making two equally spaced cuts in each direction. If in doubt, use a tape measure. Your portion size is only as accurate as the distance between your cuts! Put your piece(s) into a microwave-safe bowl.
2. *Pour your milk into a liquid measure.* Pour it into a glass to drink, use it to top your pie, or divide it between the two.
3. Heat the Multi-Grain Pie in the microwave for one to two minutes on high.
4. *Pour your juice into a liquid measure* and then into your juice glass. Note the level and try to remember it.

High-Nutrient Eating: Quick-Energy Carbs

Complex carbohydrates such as those found in grains and legumes form the backbone of a healthy diet. They're the ground floor of the USDA Food Guide Pyramid and contribute about 60 percent of the energy to the portion savvy meal plan. A great source of almost instant energy, complex carbs wake up your metabolism in the morning by breaking down into blood glucose quickly—but not so fast that they cause the rush and subsequent letdown that simple carbohydrates such as table sugar can. Complex carbohydrates would rather be burned as energy than stored as fat, and this kind of fuel is just what your body craves after fasting all night.

When you breakfast on a carb-rich dish such as Multi-Grain Pie, you'll catapult to peak morning productivity—and because these are whole grains, you also reap the benefits of fiber, vitamin E, B vitamins, and other life-extending nutrients such as magnesium, selenium, copper, manganese, and phenolic acids. Watch out, world!

CARBOHYDRATES AND BLOOD SUGAR: A HEALTHY RELATIONSHIP

Carbohydrates are the body's principal source of blood glucose, which feeds the brain, fuels the central nervous system, and powers fat metabolism. Many recent diets have recommended severely restricting carbohydrates, which spells trouble for all the important systems relying on blood glucose for their fuel. Depriving yourself of the carbohydrate energy you need can seriously impair your performance, from the office to the playing field, and can ultimately lead to hypoglycemia, a potentially dangerous blood sugar deficit characterized by feelings of hunger, dizziness, anxiety, and fatigue. Have you experienced some of these symptoms on a high-protein diet? The cure is as close as a dose of low-fat, fiber-filled, satisfying carbs.

Savvy Kitchen Strategy: Casserole Control

Casseroles are a convenient way to cook and portion food—but their size can tempt you to dip back in for seconds if you don't take charge.

Whenever you bake a casserole, whether this breakfast pie or a lasagna, immediately cut it into the number of pieces specified by the recipe. Set aside the servings you need for the coming meal. As soon as the casserole is cool (and before you sit down to your meal unless you're eating it hot from the oven), wrap each extra piece individually, place in a freezer bag, and freeze. Now you can enjoy your portion without risk of return!

BREAKFAST OUT

A leisurely breakfast out can be a great weekend pleasure. Most restaurant breakfasts are also caloric minefields, so keep your portion savvy engaged by following the same guidelines you do at home. Choose from:

➤ Cereal, nonfat milk, and juice. Order the smallest juice, and if it's still huge, ask for an extra glass and split it with a companion.
➤ Half a bagel (whole for PS 3), an English muffin, or toast (1 slice per PS level) with jam, the smallest juice, and cappuccino with nonfat milk.
➤ An egg-white or egg-substitute omelet, made according to your portions listed in Day 3, toast, and the smallest juice.
➤ Fruit plate with nonfat yogurt; give half the fruit to someone else at the table or take it home.
➤ A small fruit shake.

Space out the meal by sipping on a pot of herbal tea. Enjoy the company, and look forward to a wonderful day off fueled by your right-size meal.

Portion Savvy Empowerment: Why Commit?

Why commit to portion savvy? Because:

➤ It can change your life.
➤ It could save your life.
➤ You deserve to be as smart in your eating choices as you are in other areas of your life.
➤ Energy balance is beautiful.
➤ Once you learn, you'll be portion savvy forever.
➤ Sizing your portions to your energy needs is the only proven way to achieve and maintain a fit weight.

You take it from there.

WEEK TWO: CHALLENGE

LUNCH

The midday meal is an essential recharge, and the busier you are, the more important it is. One of my firm portion savvy principles is that you must not skip lunch! But it can be a **challenge** to eat right when you're on the go—in restaurants, at the office, in the car with the kids—and the only solution is to have a plan. This week, you'll learn how to enjoy a delicious meal in the middle of a busy day that energizes you to sail right by the afternoon slump and pack in everything you have planned, including some new portion savvy skills.

Week Two Game Plan

➤ First thing Monday morning, assess your progress (see below). Part of clicking in is getting in touch with your body, and your weekly checkup is an essential part of the process. Compare your results with last week's numbers; remember that you're starting slowly with the small steps that lead to success; and be aware that even if bodily changes seem invisible at this early stage, your mind is transforming at an amazing rate.

➤ Repeat your portion savvy breakfasts from Week One, continuing to measure your portions but focusing more on memorizing your right-size servings by sight. Think of *mental monitoring* as you serve these meals.

➤ Prepare and portion your lunches according to the following plan.

➤ At dinner, continue to cut out bread, dessert, and added fats.

➤ Eat your designated number of snacks between meals (see the Portion Savvy Snack List on pages 210 and 211).

➤ Transition into the Week Two exercise plan.

➤ Continue with your food journal, scrapbook, and rewards for the days you stick to the Portion Savvy Plan.

➤ Seek all the support you need in what many people find to be the most difficult week in establishing a new healthy habit!

ASSESS YOUR PROGRESS

➤ Refer to the instructions on page 59 for the self-assessments below.

➤ Goals can shift as you change, and your weight loss goal might alter as you become portion savvy. That's why I ask you to write it down every week after taking some time to assess your progress and decide whether your old goal still makes sense.

Weight _____

Clothes fit test (check any that are looser or fill in your new size):
_____ Pants _____ Skirt _____ Shirt or blouse _____ Blazer or jacket

Present weight goal range _____

WORKOUT: WEEK TWO

It's time to turn up the heat on the output side of your energy equation! This is a crucial week for tricking your metabolism out of its instinct to respond to your calorie cuts by moving more slowly. It's also a key moment in your motivational flow, and moving on the physical level can keep you going forward mentally and emotionally, as well as generate endorphins for a much needed natural high.

Portion Savvy Workout, Week Two

This week, your goal is to burn 300 calories a day, five days of the week. This will mean increasing your workout time from last week—for instance, you'll need to extend the 45-minute power walk that burned 200 calories to about 65 minutes to reach your new 300-calorie goal, or make sure your tennis game lasts at least 40 minutes. This is a good opportunity to expand your exercise repertoire to enjoy the fun and added benefits of cross-training—so refer to the chart on page 62 and the one below, and mix and match to your heart's content!

Exercise	Calories Burned per Half Hour*
Swimming laps	270
Water aerobics	140
Bicycling	200
Yoga	140

* By a 150-pound person.[33]

Remember that the weight-bearing exercises listed in Week One deliver the biggest fat-burning payoff if you're carrying many extra pounds—but the more you work out, the more important it is that you rotate activities to prevent injury.

MONDAY, DAY 8: PASTA, THE PORTION NEMESIS

Some form of pasta is found in nearly every world cuisine, and recent scientific discoveries that we should be eating more carbohydrates and less meat and fat have united with culinary trends to support a surge in pasta's popularity in America. Theoretically, this is good, but in practice, too much pasta is adding pounds to the population.

Contrary to some recent theories, carbohydrates such as pasta don't make you fat biochemically. But carbohydrate calories add up much faster than most people think, and extra calories do feed your fat stores. Today, you'll get a handle on this portion problem food.

BEFORE-AND-AFTER PASTA

Many people are used to using a half box of pasta as a portion. Most boxes of pasta are 12 or 16 ounces and should feed as many as eight people! Your first encounter with your right-size pasta serving might be a bit of a shock—but once you experience the pleasure of finishing a pasta meal without a bloated potbelly, you'll appreciate the power of portion control.

Because different pasta shapes yield different cooked quantities (angel-hair packs itself densely into the cup, but penne tubes take up a lot of space with air), the most accurate way to measure pasta is by its dry, precooked weight. But what if you're cooking for a group or eating leftovers? The second-best way to gauge pasta is by placing the cooked product in a dry measuring cup. Use these yield equivalents when portioning cooked pasta:

	Dry Weight	Cooked Yield
PS 1	2 oz.	1 c.
PS 2	3 oz.	1½ c.
PS 3	3½ oz.	1¾ c.

Lunch, Day 8	PS 1	PS 2	PS 3
Pasta (dry weight)	2 oz.	3 oz.	3½ oz.
Fat-free or low-fat bottled tomato sauce			
OR House Marinara*	¾ c.	1 c.	1¼ c.
Grated Parmesan cheese	1 t.	2 t.	1 T.
Mixed greens	Unlimited	Unlimited	Unlimited
Fat-free salad dressing	2 T.	2 T.	2 T.
Calories	**310**	**440**	**528**

* See the Portion Savvy Recipes beginning on page 157.

Hands-On

1. Bring a pot of water to a boil. *Place a bowl on the scale, turn the knob to zero, and add dry pasta up to the weight of your portion.* Cook pasta according to package directions and drain. Serve onto a small plate or into a shallow bowl, look at it, and store a snapshot of your portion size in your mind's eye.

2. Meanwhile, *pour the marinara sauce into a liquid measuring cup.* Heat the sauce in the microwave or in a small pan on the stove. Top the hot pasta with the sauce.
3. *Measure the Parmesan cheese with a teaspoon or tablespoon,* shake to level, and sprinkle over the pasta.
4. *Measure the salad dressing with a tablespoon* and toss with the greens. Note that even fat-free dressing contains calories and needs to be portioned!

High-Nutrient Eating: Tomato Sauce, Nectar of the Gods

The Italians not only know how to live, but they also know how to live longer with lower cancer rates, and researchers believe that the tomato sauce so common to Italian cuisine might be partly responsible for this national advantage.[34] It turns out that tomatoes are the world's best source of lycopene, a hydrocarbon carotenoid that works as an antioxidant to neutralize free radicals in the body, and they also supply the anticarcinogens p-coumaric and chlorogenic acids.

A tomato-based sauce such as a classic marinara boasts the goodness of garlic, which could lower cholesterol and blood pressure, and onions, which, like garlic, provide cancer-fighting allium. In addition to its impressive nutritional profile, tomato sauce stands in for fatty pasta toppings such as cream sauces, oil, and cheese. All of these attributes make pasta marinara a supermeal.

Savvy Kitchen Strategy: Freezing Sauces

Nothing enlivens low-fat cooking more than flavorful homemade sauces—and nothing speeds up prep more than having them on hand in the freezer. When you make the House Marinara and other sauces in this book, cook up some extra and portion your serving size directly into small, resealable freezer bags. Label and date with a waterproof marker and freeze. At mealtime, simply place your bag of frozen sauce in a bowl to prevent spills and burns, prick with a fork, pop it into the microwave, and cook on defrost for 3–5 minutes. Finish on high until heated through, 2–3 minutes.

Take a shortcut with the many good fat-free and low-fat bottled tomato sauces available in the supermarket. Look for brands with no more than 50 calories and 3 grams of fat per ½-cup serving.

Portion Savvy Empowerment: Rewrite Your Beliefs

You probably had certain beliefs about your relationship with food before you knew all the details about why it's instinctually and socially natural to overeat—and why it threatens your health and life to do so. Some of these beliefs may have been strong or broad enough to influence your entire sense of self. Think about what beliefs shaped your self-image before you made the commitment to becoming portion savvy. Write them down.

Now that you've made the commitment to change your behaviors and accepted the daily challenge that commitment entails, examine your old beliefs about your essential nature and your potential. Rewrite any that no longer work.

TUESDAY, DAY 9: SAVVY SALAD

Though salads may symbolize a healthy diet, salad dressing contributes more calories than any other food to the average American woman's diet. Something doesn't compute! Here's how to make a satisfying main-dish salad without falling into the fat trap.

Lunch, Day 9	PS 1	PS 2	PS 3
Mixed greens	2 c.	2 c.	2½ c.
Assorted chopped vegetables	1 c.	1 c.	1¼ c.
Fat-free dressing			
OR any Portion Savvy Recipe dressing*	2 T.	3 T.	4 T.
Cooked skinless chicken or turkey breast,			
shrimp, or fish	4 oz.	5 oz.	6 oz.

Fresh fruit	1 med.	1 med.	1 med.
Calories	**325**	**450**	**515**

* See the Portion Savvy Recipes beginning on page 157.
For vegetarian alternatives, see page 209.

Hands-On

1. *Use a dry measuring cup to measure the greens and chopped vegetables.* Place in a medium bowl.
2. *Measure one tablespoon of dressing,* add it to the greens and vegetables, and toss. Arrange the salad on a plate.
3. *Weigh the meat or seafood on the scale.* Slice and arrange on top of the salad.
4. *Use a tablespoon to measure the remainder of your dressing portion* and drizzle over the salad. Sprinkle with freshly ground pepper to taste.
5. *Use the portion savvy pop-out to size your fruit.*

If you prefer a chopped salad, chop the greens first (romaine works best). Weigh and chop the meat or seafood, add it to the bowl with the greens and vegetables, and toss with your entire portion of dressing.

High-Nutrient Eating: Fabulous Phytochemicals

Vegetables just couldn't be any better! In addition to offering flavor and fiber at a low calorie cost, your veggie friends are packed with phytochemicals, a broad array of vitamins and compounds that prevent disease and extend longevity. Phytochemicals can disarm cancer cells, neutralize free radicals, prevent the oxidation of fats in the bloodstream, and bind with cholesterol to remove it from the body. Scientists are only beginning to identify the individual soldiers in this antiaging army, but what's clear is that the more vegetables you eat, the more phytochemicals you get, probably including many that aren't in vitamin supplements because we haven't discovered them yet.

Eating vegetables is a big, capital-letter DO!

Savvy Kitchen Strategy: The Well-Dressed Salad

With regular salad dressing so shockingly high in fat and calories (100 calories and 10 grams of fat in a tablespoon of a simple vinaigrette), it's a shame that so many of the commercial fat-free brands are equally high in sodium or sugar, or simply taste bad. When it comes to a dressing that will have you drooling over your salad without worrying about the bad stuff, my advice is to make your own.

Every weekend, mix up a batch of salad dressing from one of the recipes in this book. Keep it in the refrigerator and use it for your main course and side salads all week long. Rotate recipes every week so you don't get bored. Your salad may be dressed to kill, but it won't hurt *you*.

Portion Savvy Empowerment: Rebel Yell

As with most learning processes, there will probably come a period during the 30-Day Plan during which you become bored, frustrated, wanting to rebel—craving a sandwich just because your meal plan says salad. Acknowledge your rebellion, confusion, boredom, or lapse of faith—and let it go.

It's exactly when it doesn't seem worth the effort that your efforts matter the most. Transitional periods of apathy, frustration, or hopelessness are natural and temporary, and psychologists believe they actually provide the downtime necessary for you to accept change into your life. Resistance and obstacles are signs that you're learning and growing at a serious, deep level. Force creates counterforce, so expect some protests from your mind and body. Your organism is designed to protect the status quo, but one of the transcendent powers of being human is the ability to change.

When times get tough, get going. Write down your feelings in your journal to help you process them and put things into perspective. Then, forge ahead! A breakthrough is right around the corner. Your temptation or despair will be swept away by a wave of new energy to pursue and achieve your goals.

All you need now is an ounce of faith. Weigh it on your kitchen scale and toss it with your salad. It enhances every flavor and is calorie free.

WEDNESDAY, DAY 10: SOUP'S ON

A pot of soup simmering on the stove symbolizes home, hearth, and nurturing. Soup can be good food and a superconvenient lunch when you serve it up portion savvy style.

Lunch, Day 10	PS 1	PS 2	PS 3
Canned fat-free soup			
(not condensed)	1 16-oz. can	1 16-oz. can	1 16-oz. can
OR Minestrone*	2 c.	2 c.	2 c.
Grated Parmesan cheese	1 t.	2 t.	1 T.
Bread or roll	1 oz.	2 oz.	2 oz.
Fresh fruit	—	—	1 med.
Calories	305	410	498

* See the Portion Savvy Recipes beginning on page 157.

Hands-On

1. *Ladle Minestrone into a 2-cup liquid measure or check the nutrition label on your canned soup.* The label should indicate no more than 100 calories and 480 milligrams of sodium per 1-cup serving; your portion is the whole can. Pour the soup into a microwave-safe bowl or a saucepan and heat in the microwave or on the stove.

2. *Measure the Parmesan cheese with a teaspoon or tablespoon;* shake to level. Sprinkle over the hot soup.
3. *Weigh your bread or roll,* and if necessary, cut it down to size.
4. *Apply the portion savvy pop-out to your fruit* (PS 3) and trim as necessary.

High-Nutrient Eating: Less Salt, More Substance

Packaged foods are the number one source of sodium in the American diet, and we're currently overdosing on salt to the tune of 4,000 milligrams a day versus the 2,400-milligram limit recommended by the federal government. This excess translates to an estimated 16 percent of the heart disease and 23 percent of the stroke deaths in people ages 25 to 55.[35]

A leading sodium offender has traditionally been canned soups, primarily because they've contained so few flavorful ingredients that the penny-pinching food industry has compensated for the shortfall with salt. But a new breed of health-conscious soups have trimmed the sodium without sacrificing flavor by packing in tasty vegetables and herbs—and needless to say, you can do even better with fresh ingredients at home.

You generally pay for the convenience of processed food with less flavor and more salt (not to mention extra dollars), so whenever you can, make it fresh.

Savvy Kitchen Strategy: Soup

In my experience, everyone who experiences the virtues of made-from-scratch soup is a convert. The trick is simply production efficiency:

➤ Make a big batch on a weekend day when you have the leisure to chop vegetables and enjoy the savory aroma drifting from your simmering pot.
➤ Cool the soup completely, then portion 2-cup servings into Tupperware-type containers. You'll need one size bigger than

pint-size to allow for expansion in the freezer and safe reheating. Freeze.

➤ Reheat your soup in the microwave directly from the freezer. (Use a small plate underneath so you don't have to handle the hot container.) If you prefer, run hot water over the sealed container, then pop the frozen soup into a pan and heat on the stove. You can take frozen soup to the office and let it sit all morning without refrigeration. It's self-cooling!

NO FREE LUNCH

Psychologists agree that everybody eats more when confronted with free food. In one experiment, college students were shown to consume about double their usual intake (1,200–1,400 calories versus an average of 700) when lunch was free. Similar cases of uncommon consumption have been observed at happy hours, salad bars, all-you-can-eat buffets, and parties across the country and the socioeconomic spectrum.

You pay the price for a free lunch with fat on your body. So the next time someone says, "I'll buy you lunch," put your portion perception in charge of your bargain-hunting instinct. As far as your body is concerned, there *is* no free lunch.

Portion Savvy Empowerment: Just Say No

This month, give yourself a break from the environmental triggers that could derail you during a delicate, formative time. Feel free to turn down social invitations that you fear might pull you off track. Stay out of restaurants if they wave a red danger flag. (Successful dieters at the National Weight Control Registry ate out no more than three times a week—twice or less in full-service restaurants, and less than once in fast-food joints.) Don't dine with people who pressure you to eat more than you need. It's only a month. You'll reintegrate these activities into your life once your habits are firmly in place. Do what you need to meet your challenge in the present, and the future will take care of itself.

THURSDAY, DAY 11: THE CLASSIC SANDWICH

The sandwich is a worldwide classic, and the concept of protein and vegetables enclosed in bread is both nutritionally balanced and pragmatic. And yet this is the culinary creation that inspired the term *overstuffed.* Here's how to unstuff your sandwich and your stomach for a life-supporting lunch.

Lunch, Day 11	PS 1	PS 2	PS 3
Bread	2 oz.	2 oz.	2 oz.
Cooked turkey or chicken breast or other low-fat lunch meat	3 oz.	3 oz.	4 oz.
OR low-fat cheese (mozzarella, provolone, goat, feta, soy)	1 oz.	1½ oz.	2 oz.
Lettuce, tomato, onion, sprouts, mustard, horseradish	Unlimited	Unlimited	Unlimited
Fat-free mayonnaise, barbecue sauce, ketchup	Up to 1 T.	Up to 1 T.	Up to 2 T.
Fresh fruit	—	1 med.	1 med.
Calories	**315**	**420**	**550**

Hands-On

1. *Check your bread on the scale.* Trim slices, pita bread, English muffins, bagels, and sandwich rolls as necessary. If you like a multidecker, club-style sandwich, try extra-thin slices—weighed on the scale of course! Toast your bread if you like.
2. *Weigh your meat or cheese.* Slice if necessary.
3. Assemble your sandwich with vegetables and fat-free condiments of choice. Cut it diagonally into quarters for visual appeal and slower eating.

High-Nutrient Eating: Balancing Proportions

There's a version of the sandwich in most cuisines, and for many good reasons. Bread is an economical staple food that also happens to make a great holder for other foods to create a self-contained and portable meal. Because you can put anything inside, sandwiches invite creativity and individual choice. But most important, the combination of bread, meat, and vegetables that typically comprises the sandwich can be perfectly balanced from a nutritional standpoint. The carbohydrates generate energy for a midday recharge, the protein provides staying power and releases alertness chemicals to keep you sharp through the afternoon slump, and the vegetables fill in vitamins and fiber.

In most other cultures, sandwiches are slim. Unfortunately, many American sandwiches subscribe to the theory that what you can't see underneath the bread—thick slabs of meat, mayonnaise, cheese, dressing, oil—won't hurt you. But it will. *A national survey of deli sandwiches found that the average overstuffed tuna salad sandwich weighs in at 857 calories and 50 grams of fat. A Reuben racks up the same amount of fat and 916 calories.* Don't think you're being virtuous if you order vegetarian; that route will cost you 753 calories and 40 grams of fat.[36] How did we get into this predicament? As we are prone to do, Americans took a good idea and went hog-wild.

Remember this: A properly proportioned sandwich is compact and doesn't drip. It respects the beauty of its balance and fits as easily into your mouth as it does into your shrinking stomach.

Savvy Kitchen Strategy: Meat Made Easy

When it comes to portioning your sandwich meat, you can let other people do the work for you. At the supermarket deli, ask your server to slice your meat thin, weigh it, and wrap it in individual packets of your portion size (3 or 4 ounces). If you prefer to purchase packaged lunch meat, choose the low-fat brands and read the label. Most will tell you how many slices are in a 2-ounce serving; cut that number in half for the slices in an ounce, multiply it by 3 or 4 (PS 1, 2, or 3), and that's how many slices go in your sandwich.

Portion Savvy Empowerment: Assertive Visualization

Portion savvy people control their environments, not vice versa. Paradoxically, control of your external circumstances comes not from the outside but from within, and assertive visualization is an effective tool for managing any situation you might encounter.

Get into the habit of visualizing yourself in the world being and behaving exactly as you want to be. Before a party, picture yourself in your best outfit looking gorgeous, conversing easily and pleasurably, sipping on some sparkling water, and eating the portions you had planned for your beautiful body. Prepare for a presentation or interview by playing out the scene in your mind—what you'll wear, what you'll say, and a nonfood way to celebrate your success. Picture yourself portioning your plate one month from now. It's easy and automatic, like brushing your teeth.

Practice makes perfect, and when you control your environment through visualization, you'll see barriers melt away, doubts and fears dissolve, and empowerment become yours.

FRIDAY, DAY 12: THE BURRITO BOMBSHELL

Burritos are the original wrap—and a longtime favorite at Diet Designs because they're as adventurous as they are satisfying. Most burritos sink like the *Titanic* in your stomach and are equally catastrophic in caloric terms . . . but not the portion savvy kind.

Lunch, Day 12	PS 1	PS 2	PS 3
Cooked beans (pinto, kidney, black, lentils, etc.)	½ c.	¾ c.	¾ c.
Cooked brown rice	⅓ c.	½ c.	¾ c.
Salsa	Unlimited	Unlimited	Unlimited

Low-fat tortilla	1 8-inch	1 10-inch	1 10-inch
Grated low-fat cheddar cheese	1 T.	1 T.	1 T.
Fat-free sour cream	1 T.	1 T.	1 T.
OR Vegetarian Burrito*	PS 1	PS 2	PS 3
Calories	**329**	**435**	**518**

* See the Portion Savvy Recipes beginning on page 157.

Hands-On

1. *Measure the beans and then the rice in dry measuring cups for your PS level.* Combine in a small bowl, warm in the microwave or on the stovetop, and mix with salsa to taste.
2. Warm the tortilla for 30 seconds under the broiler or wrapped in plastic in the microwave. Spoon the bean and rice mixture over the bottom third.
3. *Measure the cheese with a tablespoon, packing and leveling with your fingers.* Sprinkle over the bean mixture.
4. Fold in the ends of the tortilla and roll up.
5. *Measure the sour cream with a tablespoon, leveling with a knife.* Dollop over the burrito and serve with additional salsa as desired.

High-Nutrient Eating: Legumes for Life

Quick: What costs just pennies per serving, lowers cholesterol, is packed with low-fat protein and high-energy carbohydrates, contains a blood-pressure-lowering cocktail of calcium and potassium, and ices the cake with B vitamins, iron, potassium, and magnesium? It's beautiful beans! Pintos; kidneys; black, white, red, and pink; limas and lentils; garbanzos and great northerns; black-eyed peas and navy beans—the list goes on. Beans set the standard for healthy, high-nutrient eating, and their value doubles when they stand in for some of the meat in your diet.

If you had to pick a fight with beans, the only thing you could complain about is their lack of methionine, one of the nine essential amino acids needed to provide complete protein to the body. But this is splitting hairs, because you can make up the difference by eating some grains during the same day (such as the rice and the flour tortilla in a burrito). Now your protein is perfect.

Like most carbohydrate-rich foods, beans jam a lot of calories into a small space—about 230 in a 1-cup serving. So don't mess with beans without a measuring cup.

Savvy Kitchen Strategy: Bean Basics

Cooking beans requires a little time, but no particular talent. Here are some general guidelines.

	Dry Quantity	Water	Procedure	Yield
Beans	1 lb.	6 cups	Bring to a boil, reduce heat, and simmer, partially covered, until tender.	5 c.
Brown rice	1 c.	2½ c.	Bring to a boil, stir, reduce heat, and simmer, covered, 45–50 minutes.	3–4 c.

Canned beans are fine when you don't want to cook! Drain and rinse them to lower the sodium count. If beans tend to be noisy in your digestive tract, try a squirt of Beano on your first bite. It works!

Portion Savvy Empowerment: Fun with—and without—Food

DANGER ZONE! My practice has shown that the weekend of the second week is a common time to get off track in a new eating plan. The National Center for Health Statistics has found that Americans eat the most over the weekend.[37] Challenge yourself to beat the odds. And now, have fun.

Don't agonize over the ounces. Instead, focus on how clever you are to outwit that mammoth bagel, what a blast it is to eat a burrito without feeling a thousand pounds heavier, what sensuous pleasure a perfectly grilled burger can bring.

Smile. The simple act of turning up the corners of your mouth can have a powerful effect on your emotions and outlook—so this weekend, make a point of smiling throughout your meals. Have a smile in between bites. Laugh at funny things people say. Use a smile to let your mind and body know how happy you are about your new eating plan. It could even improve your digestion!

Take the weekend to inventory all the ways you like to have fun that don't involve food. Write them down in your journal. Schedule them more frequently.

SATURDAY, DAY 13: THE GOOD BURGER

There's nothing like a Saturday to make you want to kick back with a burger. Go ahead, fire up the barbie. You've worked hard and you deserve a little play!

Lunch, Day 13	PS 1	PS 2	PS 3
Ground turkey or chicken breast, salmon, lean beef, or soy burger mixture (raw) OR BBQ Chicken, Salmon, or Soy Burger*	4 oz.	6 oz.	8 oz.
Bun, bread, or English muffin	1½ oz.	2 oz.	2 oz.
Lettuce, tomato, onion, mustard, pickles	Unlimited	Unlimited	Unlimited
Fat-free mayonnaise, ketchup, relish	Up to 1 T.	Up to 1 T.	Up to 2 T.
Jicama Slaw*	½ c.	½ c.	½ c.
Calories	**345**	**450**	**510**

* See the Portion Savvy Recipes beginning on page 157.

Hands-On

➤ Try light buns or English muffins to hold your burger with minimal weight.

1. *Place a small bowl on the scale and turn the knob to zero. Add ground turkey, chicken, salmon, or soy mixture to your PS weight.* Season to taste and form into a patty.
2. Grill, broil, or sauté burger in a nonstick pan until cooked through, about 3–5 minutes per side. (Or see the directions in the Portion Savvy Recipes.)
3. Meanwhile, *check your bun on the scale.* If it's over your PS weight, discard half or hollow it out until you reach your target weight.
4. *Measure the Jicama Slaw with a dry measuring cup;* level off.
5. Place the burger on the bun and add specified condiments to taste.

High-Nutrient Eating: Betterburger versus Badburger

While there's nothing nutritionally wrong with a ground-meat patty on a bun, Americans have developed a taste for big, fat badburgers dripping with cheese and dressing that has put the typical version of the dish off limits for health-conscious people. *A 7-ounce beef burger with 2 ounces of cheddar cheese and 2 tablespoons of Thousand Island dressing on a 2-ounce bun contains 1,200 calories and 80 grams of fat—and we haven't even added avocado or bacon yet!* At many restaurants, especially fast-food outlets, the sodium might kill you before the saturated fat even has a chance to settle on your arterial walls.

Enter the betterburger. It's made of low-fat meat, fish, or soy; served without fatty toppings but dressed up with your choice of flavorful, fat-free condiments; and presented on a bun that doesn't overwhelm the burger. It's fast, fun, delicious, and a good balance of protein, carbohydrate, B vitamins, iron, and, if you add some sliced tomatoes, even phytochemicals!

Savvy Kitchen Strategy: The Perfect Patty

Shop your kitchenware store for a patty mold or baking ring that holds just your portion. Practice a few times by weighing the meat first and then pressing into the mold; once you're sure you've got the right size, you can skip the scale.

Save yourself some prep time by buying fresh salmon burgers at the seafood counter; weigh them before cooking and resize as necessary. If you prefer veggie burgers, check the freezer case for low-fat brands that weigh in at about 2½ ounces and 110 calories each; your portion is one burger for PS 1, one and a half for PS 2, and two for PS 3.

For the moistest and most tender burger, grind your meat or fish at home right before cooking. Weigh it, place it in the bowl of a food processor fitted with a metal blade, season to taste, and gently pulse just until ground. Do not overprocess. For a special treat, make a fresh-ground burger with sirloin steak trimmed of all visible fat. If you prefer to buy ground beef, look for meat labeled as no more than 7–15 percent fat. Remember, being portion savvy means eating the food you love!

Portion Savvy Empowerment: Body Imaging

Are you ready for the naked truth? Start your day in the buff in front of a full-length mirror. Look carefully and acceptingly at yourself. Now, take out your scrapbook and a pencil and draw an outline of your body from the front, side, and rear. Focus on seeing yourself as you really are, aiming for truth and setting any artistic hesitations aside.

You can get dressed if you like before the next step. Draw each of the three body views as you'd like to look in the future. Which specific parts and proportions do you want to change? Be realistic. This will be your body, not a new one magically conferred by a fairy godmother, but it will be tangibly transformed by your new habits. Your future physique will embody the balance of energy in and out that portion savvy achieves. Look at these images frequently and acknowledge all the positive changes in your body to guide you toward your goals.

SUNDAY, DAY 14: AN ELEGANT PASTA SALAD

A make-ahead composed salad is always welcome at lunch—easy to take on a picnic, carry to the office, or simply grab from the fridge whenever you feel like lunch on a lazy Sunday.

Lunch, Day 14	PS 1	PS 2	PS 3
Asparagus, Lima Bean,			
and Bow-Tie Pasta Salad*	1½ C.	2 C.	2½ C.
Calories	**324**	**433**	**540**

* See the Portion Savvy Recipes beginning on page 157.

Hands-On

1. *Measure your pasta salad with a dry measuring cup.*

    Easy!

High-Nutrient Eating: Plant Protein

Most Americans eat too much meat and could realize many health and energy benefits by incorporating more vegetarian meals, such as this beautifully balanced pasta salad, into their diets.

The main arguments for cutting back on meat consumption are its high saturated-fat content and its lack of the life-extending phytochemicals and fiber that plant foods have. The challenge with vegetarian meals is achieving adequate complete protein, which your cells need for ongoing regeneration and repair.

Your body requires nine essential amino acids from your diet to synthesize complete protein, and no plant food except soy provides the right balance of all nine. That's why the more vegetarian meals you eat, the more you should look for complementary protein combinations, food pairings that fill in each other's missing amino acids. Generally, grains complement legumes—which makes pasta and lima beans a complete protein pair—and legumes complement seeds.

You don't have to eat complementary plant foods in the same meal to get their full protein punch, but they do have to be digested within the same day—so you can simplify your record keeping with one-dish complements such as Asparagus, Lima Bean, and Bow-Tie Pasta Salad.

Savvy Kitchen Strategy: The Freezer as Flavor Arsenal

The delicious artichoke pesto that dresses today's salad is just the sort of trick that can transform a quick low-fat meal from ho-hum to special. Satisfying your taste buds is essential to staying portion savvy. Hit your palate with a zesty sauce and it will be happy with much less pasta.

But everyone needs a time-saver when it comes to flavor, and here's today's: Make a double batch of the artichoke pesto for this recipe. Freeze it in your PS portion in small resealable freezer bags, and use it to top chicken and fish (which you'll learn about next week). Think of flavor as your secret weapon in the fight against fat, and your freezer is where you store your stash.

Portion Savvy Empowerment: You Rule!

CONGRATULATIONS!

You've made it through the challenge week, the hardest period of becoming portion savvy. Give yourself a huge pat on the back for being so good and relax in the knowledge that, from now on, *it just gets easier!*

OUT TO LUNCH

Here are some easy ways to stay savvy when lunch is out and about.

The Savvy Salad Bar

Salad bars can be a great source of phytochemicals on the go, but the combination of high-fat items and all-you-can-eat portions sabotages many salad bar patrons. The portion savvy strategy is to keep it simple:

➤ Choose any greens and vegetables you like. Skip anything prepared with mayonnaise or cream.

➤ Add cooked beans or cottage cheese: 2 heaping tablespoons for PS 1, 3 for PS 2, or 4 for PS 3.

➤ Top with *fat-free* dressing, or vinegar, lemon juice, and black pepper to taste.

➤ Scoot right by the nuts, fried noodles, pasta, prepared salads, soups, casseroles, and bread. When you're done, your meal should look like a salad, not a smorgasbord.

At the Deli

➤ Rule of thumb: To portion a restaurant or deli sandwich, split it with a friend or order it open-faced and remove half the filling.

➤ Portions by the pint: When you're far from your measuring cup, remember the portion power of the deli tub. Half-pint deli containers (they're the low, flat ones) hold one cup; one-pint tubs hold two cups. With these benchmarks and today's portions as your gauge, you can order a grain-and-bean salad with low-fat dressing at any deli.

Defusing the Burrito Bombshell

You can enjoy a restaurant burrito *if* you employ these bomb squad tactics:

➤ Order it with rice, beans, and salsa; *low-fat* cheese or sour cream only (follow your portion guidelines); no meat. Add chopped onion, hot peppers, and additional salsa to taste.

➤ If you're PS 1, cut the burrito in half and give the rest away or take it home. PS 2 can eat three-quarters, and PS 3 gets the whole thing.

➤ Skip the chips on the side. They're loaded with fat and sodium.

WEEK THREE: CONCENTRATION

Dinner

The last meal of the day can be a rewarding family experience, a time to relax, and an opportunity to focus on the pleasures of the table—but it's also by far the most common meal for overeating. This week, you're going to align your dinner with your dietary needs; examine your feelings about food, family, and reward; and enjoy some delicious meals that fulfill my promise that portion savvy is a delicious and satisfying way of life.

You've made the commitment and accepted the challenge; now, **concentrate** on applying what you've learned in the past two weeks to perfect your portioning skills.

Week Three Game Plan

➤ Begin the week by assessing your progress.
➤ Repeat the meal plans from Week One for breakfast and Week Two for lunch; follow the instructions in this chapter for dinner.
➤ Eat your designated number of snacks between meals (see the Portion Savvy Snack List on pages 210 and 211).
➤ Take advantage of your increasing energy levels with the Week Three workout program, which will combine with the full-day portion savvy eating plan to nudge you into the serious fat-burning zone.

➤ Continue with your food journal and scrapbook.
➤ During this week, eating and exercising according to plan should start to become its own reward. You can taper down or stop the specific daily rewards called for in the first two weeks if you like—but if they motivate or inspire you, by all means keep it going!

ASSESS YOUR PROGRESS

Refer to the instructions on page 59 for the self-assessments below.

Weight _____

Clothes fit test (check any that are looser or fill in your new size):
_____ Pants _____ Skirt _____ Shirt or blouse _____ Blazer or jacket

Present weight goal range _____

WORKOUT: WEEK THREE

This should be an exciting week for your body, in which you start to see and feel the payoff of your eating and exercise plan. You'll probably find that you're able to work out harder and longer than before and begin to notice how exercise can actually help regulate your hunger levels. Now that you're well launched on a fat-burning regime, it's time to add resistance training to your routine to build lean muscle mass, boost metabolism, and strengthen bones.

Portion Savvy Workout, Week Three

Amp up your workouts to burn 350 calories apiece, five times this week. Continue with the activities of the past two weeks (see pages 62 and 84), mixed in with two to three sessions of resistance training: weight machines, free weights, Pilates, or resistance bands.

Exercise	Calories Burned per Half Hour*
Weight lifting, light to moderate	100

* By a 150-pound person.[38]

Try a 50-minute bike ride, half an hour of lap swimming followed by half an hour of weight machines, an hour-long aerobics class including 15 minutes with resistance bands or free weights, an hour of heavy yard work, or 45 minutes on the soccer field to burn those 350 calories. It's always a good idea to warm up for resistance-training sessions with a cardiovascular activity, which will also help you get to your energy expenditure goal faster. Don't forget to stretch before and after your workout.

MONDAY, DAY 15: CHICKEN BREASTS, BASIC AND BEYOND

The introduction of boneless, skinless chicken breasts to the nation's supermarkets was a major coup for everyone who appreciates good food. They're fast, fresh, low-fat, elegant, versatile—and best of all, they're preportioned. Learn to size up and sauce a chicken breast half, and dinner is served.

Dinner, Day 15	PS 1	PS 2	PS 3
Boneless, skinless chicken breast	4 oz.	5 oz.	6 oz.
Mustard Cream Sauce*			
OR any Portion Savvy Recipe sauce*	2 T.	2 T.	3 T.
Cooked rice or grain	½ c.	¾ c.	¾ c.
Steamed or grilled vegetables	1 c.	1½ c.	1½ c.
Calories	**346**	**401**	**519**

* See the Portion Savvy Recipes beginning on page 157.
For vegetarian alternatives, see page 209.

Hands-On

1. *Place a boneless, skinless chicken breast on the scale and trim to your PS weight. Now, hold your portion savvy pop-out over the*

chicken and imprint this image in your visual memory. Save any trimmings for use in pastas, pizzas, burgers, and salads. Grill, broil, bake, or poach chicken.

2. *Measure the Mustard Cream Sauce with a tablespoon.* Top the chicken with the sauce.

3. *Measure cooked grains with the dry measuring cup(s) for your PS level.* Place your side dish on the plate alongside the chicken and *frame with the portion savvy pop-out to create a visual image of your right-size serving.*

4. *Measure the cooked vegetables with the dry measuring cup(s) appropriate to your PS level.* Serve.

High-Nutrient Eating: Protein Power

Interested in hanging on to your muscles, organs, tissues, skin, hair, fingernails—your cells themselves? Then you need protein. Specifically, you need about 0.8 grams of protein per day for each kilogram of body weight (pounds divided by 2.2), which is 58 grams for a 160-pound person. This requirement may vary with age, physical activity, pregnancy, and some medical conditions.

Lean varieties of poultry, meat, and seafood are the most calorie-efficient sources of complete protein, and the Portion Savvy Plan takes advantage of this nutritional edge with moderate servings of animal foods. But the proportion of these foods in your diet must be monitored and balanced for health and weight management. Not only are many meats high in saturated fat, but eating too much animal protein is associated with higher LDL cholesterol levels, possible increased risk of certain types of cancers, and elevated levels of homocysteine compounds that have been linked with increased risk of heart disease. The best diet for long life balances all the food groups to provide adequate protein (as well as carbohydrates, fat, vitamins, minerals, and fiber) without overloading on animal foods or calories. Tonight's dinner, which unites a right-size serving of protein with complex carbohydrates and vegetables, provides a perfect example of that magic mix.

Savvy Kitchen Strategies: Cook, Season, Portion, Eat!

Dinner should be both easy and a special time with family and friends. That's why the Portion Savvy Plan for dinner centers around quick-cooking poultry, seafood, and meat coupled with low-fat seasoning techniques. The Portion Savvy Recipes will give you plenty of ideas for sauces, marinades, and spice rubs that add flavor to your meat and seafood dishes. Once you've got the basic cook-and-season concept down and learn to add your side dish servings, dinner is a snap!

Make enough Mustard Cream Sauce to top your fish and pork tenderloin later in the week. It's only Monday, but you'll have Wednesday's and Friday's dinners almost in the bag.

If you prefer the economy of buying bone-in chicken breasts with skin, debone the breasts and remove the skin at home.

Portion Savvy Empowerment: Concentration

To concentrate is to focus on one issue at a time. Concentration sifts what's important out of all the influences and incoming messages around you and leaves the rest as background noise.

This week, filter out the other issues and activities associated with dinner while you concentrate on learning your portion sizes. If you have a family, ask your partner to stay out of the kitchen and listen to the kids' stories while you focus on mindfully managing your food. It's a small sacrifice that will pay off in a new, automatic portion sense that can stand up to the chaos of the dinner hour.

TUESDAY, DAY 16: COMFORTING CASSEROLES

Casseroles are home-cooking favorites because they're efficient, feed a family, can be made ahead, and freeze well—but they're also often high in calories and fat. In today's lesson you'll learn how to throw together a soul-satisfying lower-fat lasagna and slice it up with good portion perception.

Dinner, Day 16	PS 1	PS 2	PS 3
Polenta Lasagna*	1 piece	1½ pieces	1½ pieces
Mixed greens	Unlimited	Unlimited	Unlimited
Fat-free dressing	2 T.	2 T.	2 T.
Fruit	—	—	1 med.
Calories	**309**	**451**	**526**

* See the Portion Savvy Recipes beginning on page 157.

Hands-On

1. Prepare and bake the lasagna according to the recipe.
2. *Cut the casserole into eight pieces with three lengthwise cuts and one cut across.* Space your cuts as evenly as possible.
3. *Serve the number of pieces specified for your PS level,* accompanied by salad.

High-Nutrient Eating: Unclogged Cheese

Cheese ranks with beef and milk as one of the top three sources of saturated fat in the American diet, mostly due to our love of gooey things like lasagna and pizza. We're up to over half a pound of cheese a week per person—and if you were to look at that melted and pooled on a plate, you'd *know* you don't want it in your arteries!

But cheese is also a good source of calcium, protein, and pure comfort—so portion savvy people take a low-fat, high-flavor approach that makes a little go a long way. Today's lasagna combines tangy goat cheese (naturally low in fat), nutty Parmesan (very flavorful), and fat-free mozzarella to give you a light and tasty *fromage* fix. Take tonight to focus on the pleasure of cheese, and then remember that it should never be a careless add-on to your meals.

Savvy Kitchen Strategy: Cut 'n' Freeze

As convenient as casseroles are to make, they offer the temptation of seconds and leftovers. Avoid this risk with two savvy steps:

➤ Cut the entire casserole into portions at once, not just what you're serving. The psychological fence of portioned pieces will prevent attack by your passing fork.

➤ As soon as the lasagna is completely cool, individually wrap remaining portions in plastic and freeze immediately. Now you've got dinner for next week!

LAST-CHANCE EATING

For many people, dinner is the most emotional meal of the day. Imbued with the ideals and emotions of family time, home and hearth, dinner epitomizes the notion of sharing food as love — and more food feels like more love. It's also a natural time to reward yourself for a good day or to comfort yourself after a bad or stressful one. Supper is your last chance to eat today, and some people suffer a silent, subconscious fear that the next meal will never come.

A study measuring satiety on diets of low and high caloric density found that dinner was the one meal at which people on both diets ate to the point of discomfort.[39] My Diet Designs clients report dinner to be the most common time for slipups. Even without emotional variables, chatting with your loved ones and feeling fatigued from a full day can distract you from your best intentions, so it's crucial that you preset your portions on your dinner plate and do so repeatedly until it's simply second nature.

If you find yourself falling victim to a feeling of last-chance eating, remember that you'll eat every day for the rest of your life, starting with breakfast tomorrow.

Portion Savvy Empowerment: Mindful Eating

Tonight, try eating without conversation or the radio, television, or newspaper. Concentrate on each bite, putting down your fork after each one. Take a deep breath between bites, feeling the oxygen flow through your body to nourish it just like your food. Experience how deep inhalations of air can intensify the flavors of what you're eating and help to circulate the energy of your meal throughout your body. Note how silence provides the clear space you need for your awareness to arise.

It's too easy, in a fast-paced life filled with stimuli from every direction, to eat without thinking or even perceiving the food you ingest. Unmindful eating can lead to the habit of gulping down meals, which will blow your calorie control and disrupt your digestion. Mindful eating slows down your intake so your satiety signals can keep up and your body can rebalance in peace.

WEDNESDAY, DAY 17: THE OTHER WHITE MEAT

Tired of turkey and chicken breast? Many people don't know that pork tenderloin is just as low in fat, and it makes a delicious and easy-to-cook change of pace that lends itself to a variety of seasonings and sauces.

Dinner, Day 17	PS 1	PS 2	PS 3
Roasted pork tenderloin	4 oz.	5 oz.	6 oz.
Mustard Cream Sauce*			
OR any Portion Savvy Recipe sauce*	2 T.	2 T.	3 T.
Baked potato or yam	½ (4 oz.)	½ (4 oz.)	½ (4 oz.)
Steamed or grilled vegetables	1 C.	1½ C.	1½ C.
Calories	**380**	**434**	**503**

* See the Portion Savvy Recipes beginning on page 157.
For vegetarian alternatives, see page 209.

Hands-On

1. *Place a dinner plate on the scale and turn the knob to zero. Carve the roasted pork tenderloin into ½-inch slices and place on the plate up to your allotted weight.*
2. *Measure the Mustard Cream Sauce with a tablespoon.* Top the pork with the sauce.

3. *Return your plate to the scale, turn the knob to zero, and add your baked potato or yam; cut away the excess to reach your PS weight. Now, place your portion savvy pop-out over the potato and memorize the visual image of its size.*
4. *Measure the cooked vegetables with dry measuring cup(s) for your PS level. Serve.*

High-Nutrient Eating: One Potato Two

Potatoes and yams are a carbohydrate lover's best friend. Fat-free, filling, and far more nourishing than a refined-flour product like French bread, a baked potato is the perfect balance to a meal of meat, seafood, or poultry. No matter what color your spud, it will give you complex carbs, fiber, vitamin C, and potassium; go yellow with a yam and you'll add a whopping dose of the antioxidant vitamins A and E.

The only problem with potatoes is that they seem to grow bigger every year. Learning to portion them properly could easily save you hundreds of calories a day, so take an extra minute with your portion savvy pop-out to imprint your potato size in your mind's eye.

Savvy Kitchen Strategy: Pork

Pork tenderloin is easy to prepare, requiring just a baking dish, a hot oven, and some time. Make the sauce and side dishes while the pork roasts.

To cook a 1½-pound pork tenderloin: Preheat the oven to 350 degrees. Place the pork in a baking dish and roast for 30–40 minutes or until it reaches an internal temperature of 155 degrees. Let stand, covered, 10 minutes; slice into medallions and serve.

If you don't want to roast an entire tenderloin, cut the raw pork into medallions to grill or sauté in a nonstick pan. Freeze the remaining medallions in individual packets of your portion. Defrost before cooking.

For easy potato portions, weigh your spuds at the supermarket (they should weigh 8 ounces whole; your portion is a 4-ounce half) or bring your portion savvy pop-out to the store to size up potatoes visually before you buy.

WASTE LESS, WANT LESS

It's just this side of sin for many people. It conjures up qualms from religious concerns to the primeval fear of going hungry in the future. Wasting food is an American taboo, a slap in the face to the Puritan heritage that informs all of our social practices no matter what our personal backgrounds.

As a result, we routinely waste food on our bodies. The extra body fat we carry is a sad and tangible reminder of our miscalculations.

Portion savvy people take home or give away food when it's more than they need. They send half-eaten plates back to the kitchen. At Diet Designs, we give our leftovers to a distribution program for the homeless. Identify restaurants in your community with similar programs, and dine there in confidence that your oversize portions aren't being wasted on your body or in the world.

Portion Savvy Empowerment: The Well-Dressed Plate

Food can be beautiful—so when you put your portion savvy meals on the plate, take a little extra time to make sure they're as pretty as possible.

Tonight, for instance, arrange your slices of pork tenderloin in an overlapping semicircle. Drizzle the Mustard Cream Sauce over them in a free-form, Jackson Pollock motif. Nestle your potato within the arc of the circle and sprinkle it with paprika for color. Scatter your vegetables over the rest of the plate and garnish with some fresh green herbs.

After you sit down, take a minute to look at your dinner and see what a work of art it is. You did this for *you*—and the pleasure begins even before your first bite.

THURSDAY, DAY 18: PASTA EXPRESS

Every night at dinnertime, millions of people across the country are putting pasta into a pot. Pasta is quick, satisfying, economical, and versatile. And when you learn to avoid the traps of cream, cheese, oil, and staggering portions that can plague innocent pasta, it's as healthy as can be.

Dinner, Day 18	PS 1	PS 2	PS 3
Pasta (dry weight)	1 oz.	1½ oz.	2 oz.
Fat-free or low-fat bottled tomato sauce			
OR House Marinara*			
OR chopped or sliced vegetables	¾ c.	1 c.	1½ c.
Cooked skinless chicken breast	4 oz.	5 oz.	6 oz.
OR shrimp, scallops, clams, or fish	5 oz.	6 oz.	8 oz.
Grated Parmesan cheese	1 t.	1 t.	2 t.
Mixed green salad	—	Unlimited	Unlimited
Fat-free dressing	—	2 T.	2 T.
Calories	**350**	**460**	**530**

* See the Portion Savvy Recipes beginning on page 157.
For vegetarian alternatives, see page 209.

Hands-On

1. *Place a bowl on the scale and turn the knob to zero. Add dry pasta to your PS weight.* Cook pasta according to package directions. (Or see page 85 for cooked yield equivalents.) Note that your pasta portion for this meal, which includes chicken or seafood, is smaller than for the vegetarian pasta lunch you prepared in Week Two.
2. *Weigh the cooked chicken or seafood.* Count shrimps or clams and remember their size.

COUNT YOUR SHELLFISH

Sometimes it's easier to count your shellfish than to weigh them—especially in the case of clams, whose shells mask the weight of the meat. Here's the math:

1 ounce = 1 medium shrimp
1 sea scallop
2 large clams
3 small clams

For instance, if you're in PS 1, simply count 5 medium shrimp or 15 small clams for your right-size serving.

➤ **Try linguine with clams:** Instead of red sauce, choose mushrooms, asparagus, peas, onion, garlic, and capers. Sauté in clam juice with a splash of white wine.

3. *Measure the sauce in a liquid measure or vegetables in the dry measuring cup(s) for your serving.* Heat the sauce on the stovetop or in the microwave, or sauté vegetables in chicken, vegetable, or clam broth until tender.

4. Toss together the cooked pasta, chicken or seafood, and sauce or vegetables. *Measure the Parmesan with a teaspoon and shake to level;* sprinkle over the pasta. Serve with salad.

High-Nutrient Eating: Eat Your Shellfish

Shrimp, scallops, clams, lobster, calamari—these tasty mollusks once suffered a bad reputation because, unlike their finned friends from the deep, they contain cholesterol. But the good name of shellfish has since been cleared. It turns out that the cholesterol in your blood is actually a function of how much saturated fat, not cholesterol, you eat. Shellfish register low in the saturated fat department, so you can enjoy them guilt-free—and aren't they just great with pasta?

Portion Savvy Empowerment: *Mangia!*

Many dieters make the mistake of skipping meals, believing that they're doing themselves a favor by cutting calories from their day. Nothing could be further from the truth.

When you skip a meal—whether breakfast, lunch, dinner, even a snack—you send a scarcity message to your metabolism that instructs it to burn fewer calories. You arrive at your next meal starved, your good sense goes out the door, and you overeat to compensate for your previous deprivation. Your feeding frenzy meets sluggish metabolic machinery, and the result is the conversion of excess energy to body fat.

When you follow the Portion Savvy Plan, you can eat every scheduled meal and snack with the confidence that this food provides just the calories your personal energy equation requires. There's no need to skip, and doing so could actually jeopardize your success.

FRIDAY, DAY 19: FABULOUS FISH

With an unprecedented variety of fresh fish available across the country, it's an added bonus that this nutrient-dense food is also low in calories and fat—so you get to enjoy larger servings!

Dinner, Day 19	PS 1	PS 2	PS 3
Fresh fish fillet	5 oz.	6 oz.	8 oz.
Mustard Cream Sauce*			
OR any other Portion Savvy Recipe sauce*	2 T.	2 T.	3 T.
Cooked rice or grains	½ c.	¾ c.	¾ c.
Steamed or grilled vegetables	1 c.	1½ c.	1½ c.
Calories	**356**	**456**	**529**

* See the Portion Savvy Recipes beginning on page 157.
For vegetarian alternatives, see page 209.

Hands-On

1. *Weigh your fish on the scale and trim away any excess. Now hold your portion savvy pop-out over the fillet and take a picture in your mind.* File it in the memory bank under "fish portion." (Note

that the thickness of fish fillets can vary significantly. The portion savvy pop-out is for fillets one inch thick; if your fish is thicker, the length and width of your portion savvy serving might be smaller, and vice versa. That's why the scale is so important!)

2. Season the fish to taste and grill, broil, bake, or poach as desired.

3. *Measure the Mustard Cream Sauce with a tablespoon.* Top the fish with the sauce.

4. *Use a dry measuring cup(s) to measure your side dishes of rice and vegetables.* Plate and serve.

High-Nutrient Eating: Fish for Your Ticker

When it comes to fish, fat is good! Fatty fish such as salmon contain high concentrations of omega-3 essential fatty acids, a form of polyunsaturated fat that lowers cholesterol, triglyceride, and blood pressure levels and keeps blood from clotting, thus helping to prevent hypertension, heart attack, and stroke. And there may be more. Recent studies have found that eating just one serving of fatty fish per week could reduce the risk of cardiac arrest by half, and researchers propose that this protective mechanism might be activated when omega-3s increase the levels of fatty acids in red blood cell membranes, preventing platelet aggregation, coronary spasm, and arrhythmias.[40] Meanwhile, the B vitamins in seafood offer extra protection to your heart, and you get a good dose of essential minerals and low-calorie protein.

Other fish high in omega-3s include sardines, anchovies, haddock, mackerel, bluefish, herring, trout, albacore and bluefin tuna, and lake whitefish. Get your weekly serving—it's a delicious and cost-effective form of health insurance.

Savvy Kitchen Strategy: Fish Tips

Buying the freshest fish and cooking it right is essential to its appeal.

➤ Find a fish purveyor you trust, whose wares, displayed in a single layer on clean ice, all appear moist and smell sweet. Get your fish home quickly, refrigerate it, and cook it within two days of purchase.

➤ Have your fillets cut to individual portion sizes at the fish counter.

➤ A simple citrus marinade helps keep fish moist and provides a nice counterpoint to the richness of fatty varieties such as salmon. Try squeezing fresh orange, lemon, or lime juice over fish and marinating it for five minutes before cooking.

➤ In general, cook fish about ten minutes per inch of thickness. You can broil or grill cuts that are three-quarters of an inch or thicker; protect thinner cuts by baking or poaching them. Wrapping fish in foil with a sprinkle of citrus juice or wine and baking it at 400 degrees yields moist results.

Portion Savvy Empowerment: The Joy of Food

Eating should be a sensual pleasure, and one of the great benefits of the fresh foods featured in the Portion Savvy Plan is that they can provide more pleasure per ounce than the taste-impaired processed foods that come out of packages. It might seem paradoxical, but when you really enjoy your food, you're less inclined to overeat. It's the magic of the satisfaction quotient, and you can make it work for you simply by enjoying your eating experience.

Tonight, when you sit down, take a minute to admire your food, its colors and sheen. Now close your eyes and smell deeply. Identify the distinct aromas of each item on the plate, and then how they combine.

As you cut into your food, note its texture. Does it resist or yield to your fork? Perhaps it spurts juice or gently flakes.

Now take a bite, close your eyes, chew, and taste as intently as you ever have. Identify the flavor elements of sweet, salt, sour, and bitterness. Experience the flavor filling your mouth, releasing itself from the food to bring you pleasure. Be aware as you swallow of the decision you've made to give this food to your body. Let your body give thanks for your good choice. Let your mouth smile.

SATURDAY, DAY 20: SATURDAY NIGHT PIZZA PARTY

Pizza is an ancient food that the Italians probably borrowed from the Middle Eastern custom of topping flat breads with vegetables and herbs. Unfortunately, we've added several pounds of cheese and greasy meats since then. Today's portion savvy installment teaches you how to reclaim the healthy goodness of this time-honored tradition.

Dinner, Day 20	PS 1	PS 2	PS 3
Medium 12" vegetarian pizza	1 slice	2 slices	2½ slices
OR any Portion Savvy Recipe pizza*	2 slices	3 slices	4 slices
Mixed greens	Unlimited	Unlimited	Unlimited
Fat-free dressing	2 T.	2 T.	2 T.
Calories	**275**	**400**	**525**

* See the Portion Savvy Recipes beginning on page 157.

Hands-On

1. *Cut the pizza into 8 slices (medium 12") or 6 slices (Portion Savvy Recipe) and serve your allotted slices onto a plate.* Accompany with salad.

High-Nutrient Eating

Pizza is a sound nutritional concept. Essentially an open-faced sandwich, pizza provides complex carbohydrates, vegetables, protein, and calcium all in one fun package. It's complete, it's inexpensive, and it's perfect for a Saturday night party.

But pizza presents two potential problems. The first is that America's overdeveloped fat tooth has turned what was once a thin, crackly crust topped with pristine tomatoes and olive oil into an extravaganza of thick, dense bread, oozing cheese, and fatty meats. The second problem is that we tend to lose all our portion sense when it comes to pizza, shoveling slices from the box directly into our mouths without even using a plate, then hurrying back for more as if we hadn't even eaten yet. Many people who wouldn't dream of scarfing down four full dinner plates of chicken, rice, and vegetables can eat the pizza equivalent (three to four slices with pepperoni) without thinking. And should your four slices be from a meat lover's stuffed-crust pie, that's 2,000 calories without even using a knife and fork.

Consider pizza a prime opportunity to top a small amount of toothsome crust with an abundance of vegetables. Why stop at tomato sauce when you can pile on peppers, onions, mushrooms—any vegetable you can dream up!

Savvy Kitchen Strategy: Presto Pizza

Making your own pizza can be so easy and varied that you'll wonder how you ever relied on boring, greasy takeout.

➤ Freeze extra pizza dough for next week. Defrost overnight in the refrigerator.

➤ Use bottled fat-free or low-fat marinara sauce for a shortcut topping. You can also interchange barbecue sauce, or skip the sauce and just enjoy the juicy veggies.

➤ Mix and match vegetables as much as you like. Sauté hard vegetables such as onions, peppers, mushrooms, and eggplant in chicken stock or vegetable broth, or grill them. If you're firing up the barbecue for a burger at lunch, grill your pizza vegetables then.

➤ Vary the cheese, following the amounts in the recipe and choosing from the cheeses in the guidelines on page 121.

➤ Have a pizza party in which everyone gets to choose the toppings for his or her own slices.

DINING ON THE TOWN

Enjoy dinner out with these portion savvy pointers.

Chicken

The standard restaurant serving of chicken is either half the bird or a double breast. In either case remove the skin, use your portion savvy pop-out to trim it down to half a breast, and take the rest home.

Pasta

You may recall from chapter 1 that the average restaurant serving of pasta with red sauce contains 849 calories, so you can imagine what happens when you start to add cream, butter, cheese, pancetta, and all the other high-fat ingredients that restaurants tend to sneak into their pasta dishes. Are you fully aware that a carbonara sauce consists solely of butter, eggs, cream, and bacon? Fat issues aside, think about the fact that your usual serving of pasta out on the town is more than three times as big as what PS 1 people need to balance their energy equation!

➤ Ask for a half portion with red sauce, and some chicken or seafood if you like.

➤ No cream, please; just a tiny spoonful of Parmesan cheese.

➤ Add a delicate salad on the side dressed with balsamic vinegar, Dijon mustard, and lemon juice.

Pizza

➤ If you're ordering takeout or in a restaurant, ask for a medium (12″) pie with a thin crust and all the vegetables you want, cut into 8 slices. Dab the top of the pizza with a paper towel before serving to remove extra grease.

➤ Toppings:
Yes: marinara sauce; barbecue sauce; onions, tomatoes, garlic, peppers, mushrooms, eggplant, zucchini, artichoke hearts, olives, or any other vegetable; pineapple; part-skim mozzarella, soy, goat, or feta cheese.
No: pesto sauce; other cheeses or extra cheese; pepperoni, sausage, meatballs, bacon, or other meats.

➤ Always serve your full portion of pizza (1, 2, or $2\frac{1}{2}$ slices) onto a plate. When your plate is empty, you are done.

Portion Savvy Empowerment: All or Nothing

One of the most common thinking traps that snares people in the process of change is evaluating success as all or nothing. In this perfectionist approach, you see any small slipup as negating all your previous progress and tearing down your healthy boundaries like a terrorist bomb. Eating one extra slice of pizza "blows" your diet for the day (week, month . . .) and seems to provide an excuse to move on to a quart of ice cream. If you can't have it all—perfect adherence to your plan—then you'll take nothing—rampant overeating, perhaps even to the point of self-punishment.

There's not a slice of pizza in the world that can jeopardize all the positive changes you've made over the past three weeks. If you find that one has leapt down your throat while you weren't looking, congratulate yourself for all your other good behaviors today. Think about how healthy your habits are becoming. Call the day a small step toward success.

SUNDAY, DAY 21: STEW NIGHT

Sunday is perfect for a stew. Take a leisurely afternoon to prepare the ingredients and let the aroma perfume the air with the smell of home. Tonight's stew is a special comfort-food treat made from lean beef, because part of being portion savvy is feeding your soul.

Dinner, Day 21	PS 1	PS 2	PS 3
Burgundy Beef Stew*	1½ c.	2 c.	2½ c.
Calories	**334**	**445**	**556**

* See the Portion Savvy Recipes beginning on page 157.
For vegetarian alternatives, see page 209.

Hands-On

1. *Ladle the stew into a liquid measure up to your allotted portion.* Try to include a proportional mixture of meat, vegetables, and

liquid in your serving. Transfer stew to a bowl and serve piping hot.

High-Nutrient Eating: The Beef on Red Meat

Americans consume far too much red meat, in huge and frequent portions often accompanied by copious, high-fat side dishes. This kind of habit presents a quadruple health threat in the form of artery-clogging saturated fat, an overload of calories and protein, higher levels of heart-threatening homocysteines, and increased risk of various cancers, particularly of the prostate.

But, as usual, the real culprit here isn't the food but the overindulgence. *Occasional small portions* of *lean* beef can be part of a healthy diet. Beef is a nutrient-dense source of protein, B vitamins, and minerals, especially iron. The iron in beef is in the form most easily absorbed by the body—a great tonic for menstruating women! (It is possible to overload on iron, but it's highly unlikely on the Portion Savvy Plan unless you're oversupplementing or have a rare condition called hemachromatosis.) When you prepare lean beef without fat and add the fiber, vitamins, and minerals of carrots, onions, mushrooms, and potatoes, you have some truly high-nutrient eating.

For many people, beef feeds not just the body but also the spirit, its rich nourishment providing reassurance and rejuvenation. Indulge this drive when you feel the need—and the rest of the time, I recommend making the stew with turkey or chicken breast or just vegetables instead!

Savvy Kitchen Strategy: Beef

The leanest cuts of beef include top sirloin, top round, flank steak, and filet mignon, which is what I've used for tonight's stew. If you're feeling less extravagant, substitute a more economical cut such as top round. The wonderful thing about this dish is that stewing the meat in wine makes even the toughest cuts tender and juicy without any added fat. Always be sure to trim all visible fat from beef before cooking.

Take a tip from the French, who are famous for their flavorful stews, or daubes. Make your stew a day in advance. Cool and refrigerate overnight, then reheat at serving time. This not only takes the heat off the cook, allowing you to spend your Sunday afternoon somewhere else (perhaps moving your body in the great outdoors), but also allows the flavors to fully develop and blend. Freeze leftover stew in individual portions for next week.

If you'd rather have a steak than stew, broil or grill one of the cuts named above and follow the portioning guidelines for dinner on Day 17 (pork tenderloin).

THE SATISFACTION QUOTIENT

Sometimes a smaller portion of a calorie-dense food packs more satisfaction than a reduced-fat or -calorie substitute. Half a cup of Häagen-Dazs might appease your craving more deeply than five fat-free cookies, and the occasional steak could prevent a binge after too many nights of chicken.

Portion Savvy Empowerment: Mood and Food

Depression and bad moods can lead to overeating, but feeling happy can also cause you to eat more than you'd planned. Studies of people following new, healthy eating plans have found that relapses are most likely to occur:

➤ When you're depressed and alone.
➤ When you're happy and with others.
➤ When you're very hungry.[41]

In other words, your mood is neither a safeguard against nor an excuse for overeating. You could attribute your urge for a banana split to feeling sad and lonely, but evidence suggests that feeling good could make that sundae look just as logical. Ultimately, no matter what your emotional state, your mind must be in the habit of telling your body to do the right thing.

Congratulations to you for being well on your way to establishing that healthy habit!

WEEK FOUR: CONTROL
Bringing It All Together

This is the week in which all the pieces of the portion savvy puzzle fall into place. As you repeat and reinforce the portioning behaviors you've learned over the past twenty-one days, your commitment to leading a healthier, longer, and more energized life will translate into deep and natural **control** over your food. Breakfast, lunch, and dinner all begin to interrelate and make sense. Your body and mind know what to expect. You feel the click-in as you see your servings in your mind's eye, check them quickly with a pop-out or other measuring tool, and feel their right size in your stomach. Now is the time when everything comes together.

Week Four Game Plan

➤ Assess your progress.
➤ Repeat the meal plans for breakfast, lunch, and dinner from Weeks One, Two, and Three. The instructions that follow will give you some important reminders and offer variations to keep your menus fun.
➤ Eat your designated snacks at the times that you've found work best for you. (See the Portion Savvy Snack List on pages 210 and 211.)
➤ Follow the Week Four workout program, which tips you up to peak performance level for maximum fat burning and lifelong maintenance.

➤ Continue with your food journal and scrapbook.

➤ You've worked hard to get this far, meeting your challenge to yourself to change. Now, experience and enjoy the control this work and learning have brought you. Envision yourself effortlessly portioning your meals from this moment on.

ASSESS YOUR PROGRESS

Refer to the instructions on page 59 for the self-assessments below.

Weight _____

Clothes fit test (check any that are looser or fill in your new size):
_____ Pants   _____ Skirt   _____ Shirt or blouse   _____ Blazer or jacket

Present weight goal range _____

WORKOUT: WEEK FOUR

It's here!—the 2,000-calorie-per-week workout that will melt extra fat off your body and maintain your fit physique for a lifetime. This vigorous but moderate workout optimizes the caloric burn without pushing you into fat-sparing shutdown mode, and it offers maximum benefits while remaining attainable for everyone. Physically and psychologically, a workout program like this deals a double benefit: Not only does exercising at this level tone and condition your body, but it's also been shown to fire your motivation to stick with your eating plan.

Moving according to the Week Four and Beyond workout program offers protection against a host of life-threatening diseases—and you can also safeguard your healthy eating habits.

Portion Savvy Workout, Week Four and Beyond

This week and thereafter, schedule five workouts that burn 400 calories apiece. Refer to the calorie-burning charts on pages 62, 84, and

106; aim for two to three resistance training sessions per week; and rotate your activities as much as possible for maximum cross-training benefits. A sample week could look like this:

1. Try interval training at the gym: Alternate 12-minute sessions on the treadmill and stair-stepper (two of each) with 10-minute sessions on the weight machines (three in total).
2. Warm up for an hour-long yoga class with 18 minutes on the stationary bike—or ride your bike to the yoga studio.
3. Enjoy the outdoors with a 50-minute run or an hour-and-a-half-long walk.
4. Spring-cleaning time? Spend an hour on heavy household work; later in the day, exercise for half an hour with weights or resistance bands.
5. Sneak in an hour-and-a-half-long lunch on the greens playing golf.

MONDAY, DAY 22

➤ High-fiber breakfast cereal presents an easy opportunity to get a head start on the day's fiber requirement.

Breakfast	PS 1	PS 2	PS 3
Fat-free or low-fat breakfast cereal	1 oz.	1½ oz.	2 oz.
Skim milk	¾ c.	¾ c.	1 c.
Fresh fruit	1 med.	1 med.	1 med.
Calories	**290**	**325**	**450**

➤ Pasta is a primary calorie culprit in many people's diets. Measure it!— by dry weight if possible, or cooked in cups.

Lunch			
Pasta (dry weight)	2 oz.	3 oz.	3½ oz.
Fat-free bottled tomato sauce			
OR House Marinara*	¾ c.	1 c.	1¼ c.
Grated Parmesan cheese	1 t.	2 t.	1 T.
OR Pasta with Lentil Sauce*	PS 1	PS 2	PS 3
Mixed greens	Unlimited	Unlimited	Unlimited
Fat-free salad dressing	2 T.	2 T.	2 T.
Calories	**310**	**440**	**528**

➤ Interchange sauces, rubs, and marinades from the Portion Savvy Recipes for any poultry, meat, or seafood meal.

Dinner			
Boneless, skinless chicken or turkey breast	4 oz.	5 oz.	6 oz.
Any Portion Savvy Recipe sauce*	2 T.	2 T.	3 T.
OR Greek Feta Chicken*	PS 1	PS 2	PS 3
Cooked rice or grain	½ c.	¾ c.	¾ c.
OR any Portion Savvy side dish*	PS 1	PS 2	PS 3
Steamed or grilled vegetables	1 c.	1½ c.	1½ c.
Calories	**346**	**401**	**519**

* See the Portion Savvy Recipes beginning on page 157.
For vegetarian alternatives, see page 209.

Stress and Staying Savvy

We all deal with stress in our lives, from daily events to major life crises. Many of my clients are at times unhappy at work, having relationship problems, or dealing with some other major stressor. There's always something to throw you off-balance—and many people try to rebalance with food.

Stress can threaten your newly formed healthy habits, but by now you know that true balance is achieved when the energy you put into your body matches what you put out. You can't rebalance a life problem with an unbalanced energy equation.

Fortunately, you *can* rebalance in the opposite direction. A huge number of my clients have reported to me that when they get their eating lives in order, other things follow. Committing to their goal, accepting the challenge, and exerting daily control over what they eat ends up rubbing off on other aspects of their lives, and soon they're taking positive steps at work, at home, or in their relationships.

Taking control via portion savvy can be the first step toward realizing other hopes and dreams. And that gives this plan a double payoff.

Meanwhile, your healthy diet can be a potent tool in the battle against daily stress. Here's how:

➤ Eat several mini-meals throughout the day. This helps to keep a nervous stomach calm, boosts your immune system, and provides steady energy throughout your time of trouble. The Portion Savvy Plan already calls for interval eating. During high-stress times, try cutting your lunch or dinner in half and eating it in two separate meals.

➤ Emphasize carbohydrates, which stimulate the production of serotonin, a neurotransmitter that soothes you and boosts your mood. Serotonin also keeps you feeling full, to ward off the snack attacks that frequently come with stress. The Portion Savvy Plan derives about 60 percent of its energy from carbohydrates, so you're well on your way. When the tension mounts, select carbohydrate snacks and consider substituting a pasta for a protein meal.

Portion Savvy Empowerment: The Meditative Bath

Try this self-nurturing close to a stressful day: Draw a hot bath laced with your favorite oil or bubble bath. If you like, light a candle. Climb into the tub and luxuriate in the warm, enveloping water. Experience the pure pleasure of the heat on your skin.

Don't listen to music or read during your meditative bath. Focus completely on yourself. Reflect on your day, then let your mind go.

Now, clean and with your mind clear for tomorrow, crawl into bed and sink into deep, peaceful sleep.

TUESDAY, DAY 23

➤ It might not seem filling, but fruit juice is jammed with calories! Use your special small juice glass.

Breakfast	PS 1	PS 2	PS 3
Bagel	1 OZ.	2 OZ.	2 OZ.
Fat-free cream cheese			
OR Fruit or Chive Spread*	2 T.	3 T.	3 T.
Orange, grapefruit, or tomato juice	½ c.	¾ c.	1 c.
Nonfat milk (in cappuccino)	½ c.	½ c.	1 c.
Calories	**240**	**388**	**463**

➤ Salad dressing is an easy place to trim fat and calories. Experiment with fat-free bottled dressings and the recipes in this book.

Lunch	PS 1	PS 2	PS 3
Mixed greens	2 c.	2 c.	2½ c.
Assorted chopped vegetables	1 c.	1 c.	1¼ c.
Fat-free dressing			
OR Portion Savvy Recipe dressing*	2 T.	3 T.	4 T.
Cooked skinless chicken or turkey breast, shrimp, or fish	4 oz.	5 oz.	6 oz.
OR Southwestern Chicken Salad*	PS 1	PS 2	PS 3
Fresh fruit	1 med.	1 med.	1 med.
Calories	**325**	**450**	**515**

➤ Divide and conquer casseroles by cutting them into portions right out of the oven.

Dinner	PS 1	PS 2	PS 3
Polenta Lasagna*	1 piece	1½ pieces	1½ pieces
Mixed greens	Unlimited	Unlimited	Unlimited
Fat-free salad dressing	2 T.	2 T.	2 T.
Fruit	—	—	1 med.
Calories	**309**	**451**	**526**

* See the Portion Savvy Recipes beginning on page 157.
For vegetarian alternatives, see page 209.

How Low and Slow Can You Go?
The Time-Energy Displacement Advantage

When you choose foods with fewer calories and more fiber to the ounce, you eat more slowly and are satisfied with less. One study found that when people were allowed to eat as much as they wanted, they reached satisfaction with as little as 1,500 calories a day when they ate high-fiber, low-calorie foods. But when their choices included high-fat and refined foods such as bacon and ice cream, the daily total jumped to as many as 3,000 calories. Furthermore, the low-calorie diners spent 33 percent longer enjoying their meals than the high-cal eaters did. Researchers call it *time-energy displacement,* and it's an edge that can help keep you portion savvy simply through your food selection.

Note that the time-energy displacement holds true for both obese and normal-weight people and that participants were equally pleased by both diets. So no matter what your previous habits and tastes, you can enhance your portion savvy by choosing well.[42]

CHOOSE RIGHT, EAT LESS

Eat as much as you want and rack up:

1,570 calories/day:	3,000 calories/day:
Salad with low-fat dressing	Ham
Chicken	Roast beef
Turkey	Bacon
Poached eggs or egg whites	Fried eggs
Hot cereal	French fries
Brown rice	Buttered bread
Dried beans	Buttered and creamed vegetables
Whole-grain breads and crackers	Juice
Fresh fruit	Whole milk
Fresh vegetables	Soda
Skim milk	Cake
(Average 0.7 calories per gram, 7 grams fiber per 1,000 calories)	Pie
	(Average 1.5 calories per gram, 1 gram fiber per 1,000 calories)

Portion Savvy Empowerment: Reverse Negative Ideas

Negative thoughts have a sneaky way of seeming true and inevitable. Often the result of cognitive errors such as selective thinking (obsessing over your mistakes and vulnerabilities and ignoring your achievements and strengths) or overgeneralization (taking a small incident and generalizing it to your life), negative ideas can become a bad habit. The good news is that this self-defeating pattern can be broken.

The next time a negative thought pops to mind, try a reversal as in one of the following examples:

Negative Idea	Reversal
I'm losing weight too slowly.	I'm eating lots of fruits and vegetables, and with such a healthy diet I have a long life ahead of me to attain and enjoy the body I want.
I'm not loved or appreciated.	Many people love and admire me; I just need to love myself enough to let it in.
I feel too tired to get anything done.	Going to the gym will boost my energy.
I totally blew my diet; I always do.	My diet is improving every day, and the satisfaction and energy I get from the Portion Savvy Plan usually keep me safe from temptation.
I should be doing better at my job.	I'm glad that I'm eating right, feeling good, and spending time with my family and friends—and the energy this gives me will pay off in job performance.
I'll never be thin.	Every day, I'm establishing the habits that will keep me fit for life.
My parents taught me bad eating habits.	I can teach myself to eat right.

WEDNESDAY, DAY 24

➤ **Eggs are fine if you remove the yolks or use a fat-free egg substitute.**

Breakfast	PS 1	PS 2	PS 3
Egg whites	4	6	8
OR Nonfat egg substitute	¼ c.	6 T.	½ c.
Chopped vegetables	1 c.	1 c.	1 c.
Toast	1 slice	1 slice	2 slices
Pure fruit preserves	1 t.	1 t.	2 t.
Fresh fruit	1 med.	1 med.	1 med.
Calories	**305**	**337**	**485**

➤ **Always check the nutrition label on canned soups. You're looking for no more than 100 calories and 480 milligrams of sodium per 1-cup serving; soups with high levels of fiber, vitamin A, and/or vitamin C are your best bet.**

Lunch			
Canned fat-free soup (not condensed)	1 16-oz. can	1 16-oz. can	1 16-oz. can
OR Minestrone*	2 c.	2 c.	2 c.
Grated Parmesan cheese	1 t.	2 t.	1 T.
Bread or roll	1 oz.	2 oz.	2 oz.
Fresh fruit	—	—	1 med.
Calories	**305**	**410**	**498**

➤ **Pork is a low-fat meat if you pick the tenderloin; avoid all other cuts.**

Dinner			
Roasted pork tenderloin	4 oz.	5 oz.	6 oz.
Any Portion Savvy Recipe sauce*	2 T.	2 T.	3 T.
OR Pork Marbella*	PS 1	PS 2	PS 3
Baked potato or yam	½ (4 oz.)	½ (4 oz.)	½ (4 oz.)
OR any Portion Savvy Recipe side dish	PS 1	PS 2	PS 3
Steamed or grilled vegetables	1 c.	1½ c.	1½ c.
Calories	**380**	**434**	**503**

* See the Portion Savvy Recipes beginning on page 157.
For vegetarian alternatives, see page 209.

Savvy Snacking

Snacking on schedule can keep you in control, smooth out your energy levels during stressful days, and give you a few more chances to enjoy healthy food every day. Here are some tips for better snack management:

➤ Portion your snacks as soon as you open a package. Small, resealable plastic bags keep them fresh and make them mobile.

➤ Weigh or count all your snacks according to the Portion Savvy Snack List. Use nutrition labels to see how many pieces are in a 100-calorie serving and then just count them out.

➤ Pack snacks for the office, school, carpooling, the gym, trips, or anytime you're on the go. Wrap up a single portion to take along; when it's gone, get back to your busy day!

➤ Choose a high-protein snack such as yogurt or low-fat cheese to counteract midafternoon slump (the amino acids stimulate alertness chemicals in the brain), or enjoy a carbohydrate bite such as rice cakes or chips when you're feeling stressed—the resulting hit of serotonin will help to keep you calm.

➤ You can use one of your snacks for dessert after dinner. Check out the Portion Savvy Recipes for some deliciously indulgent treats!

➤ Time snacks to see you through your personal energy slumps. It's best to establish a schedule and stick with it; your body likes to know what to expect.

➤ Remember that raw vegetables are a free food. Keep some on hand at all times—a bowl of crudités on ice in the refrigerator at home, a bag of crunchy carrots and celery for the office. Reach for your veggies anytime your mouth wants to move.

Portion Savvy Empowerment:
Break the Hand-to-Mouth Connection

Even my most self-aware clients report incidents of automatic eating, in which the hand reaches out and puts food in the mouth without consulting the brain. We're so deeply conditioned to believe that more food is better that we often don't stop to think about whether we actually want or need it.

This preprogrammed behavior can pop up at home when you come across a leftover or at the office when a coworker brings in doughnuts, and it's particularly problematic at parties, where an abundance of food and party nerves can combine to fuel a rampage of mindless munching.

One simple rule can help you break the hand-to-mouth connection: Stop and think. If you engage your mind before you fill your mouth, you give yourself a chance to make a choice. Do you really want this? Does it fit into your Portion Savvy Plan? If not, is it worth the price to your progress?

Eating should be a pleasure, but at times you must delay gratification to achieve your goals and experience greater pleasure in the future. Behavioral researchers have discovered that even rats can be trained to delay gratification when the future reward beats the fleeting pleasure of the moment.[43] Delay, and then decide. If a rodent can do it, you can too.

THURSDAY, DAY 25

	Breakfast	PS1	PS2	PS3
➤ Look for muffins made with bran and whole grains and trim your muffin to your PS weight.	Low-fat, whole-grain muffin OR Cherry–Oat Bran OR Apple-Raisin			
	Bran Muffin*	1 (3 oz.)	1 (3 oz.)	1 (3 oz.)
	Diced fresh fruit	½ c.	¾ c.	1 c.
	Low-fat cottage cheese	⅛ c.	¼ c.	¾ c.
	Calories	**310**	**358**	**473**

	Lunch			
➤ Forget the "overstuffed" sandwich. Make your own with lean meats and fat-free condiments, or order a half or an open-faced sandwich.	Bread	2 oz.	2 oz.	2 oz.
	Cooked turkey or chicken breast OR other low-fat lunch meat	3 oz.	3 oz.	4 oz.
	OR low-fat cheese (mozzarella, provolone)	1 oz.	1½ oz.	2 oz.
	Lettuce, tomato, onion, sprouts, mustard, horseradish	Unlimited	Unlimited	Unlimited
	Fat-free mayonnaise, barbecue sauce, ketchup	Up to 1 T.	Up to 1 T.	Up to 2 T.
	Fresh fruit	—	1 med.	1 med.
	Calories	**315**	**420**	**550**

	Dinner			
➤ To order pasta in a restaurant, ask for a half portion with red sauce; add chicken or seafood if you like. Skip the bread and have a salad instead.	Pasta (dry weight)	1 oz.	1½ oz.	2 oz.
	Fat-free bottled tomato sauce OR House Marinara* OR chopped or sliced vegetables	¾ c.	1 c.	1½ c.
	Cooked skinless chicken breast	4 oz.	5 oz.	6 oz.
	OR shrimp, scallops, clams, or fish	5 oz.	6 oz.	8 oz.

Grated Parmesan cheese	1 t.	1 t.	2 t.
OR Turkey Tetrazzini*	PS 1	PS 2	PS 3
Mixed greens	—	Unlimited	Unlimited
Fat-free salad dressing	—	2 T.	2 T.
Calories	**350**	**460**	**530**

* See the Portion Savvy Recipes beginning on page 157.
For vegetarian alternatives, see page 209.

Special Indulgences

One of my clients came to me with what seemed like an unsolvable problem: He was scheduled to travel to Boston. Living in Los Angeles, he didn't often get to Boston, and what he wanted—what, in fact, he knew he was going to have no matter what I said—was a lobster dinner with drawn butter. Could this situation be saved?

Certainly, I said, with a little portion savvy. I told him to skip the 6-pound monster lobsters and ask for a 3-pound one instead. This would yield about 16 ounces of meat to split with his dining companion. He could have two tablespoons of melted butter—measured with his spoon at the table, please!—then switch to cocktail sauce. And there should be no other saturated fat that day, which meant a vegetarian pasta lunch.

Sometimes you need to treat yourself. Deprivation isn't healthy, sustainable, or included in the meaning of *diet*. Many treats can be built into your Portion Savvy Plan, such as the fat-free Caramel Bars you can enjoy as a snack. But when you need to bend the rules, follow these principles:

➤ Plan your indulgence in advance. Special treats shouldn't be eaten on impulse.
➤ Preset the portion of your treat. Use nutrition labels, your portion savvy skills, and reasonable judgment to ensure that you're just flexing the rules lightly, not bending them out of recognizable shape.

➤ Compensate for extra fat and calories by trimming portions slightly elsewhere in your day.

Portion Savvy Empowerment: Take It Easy

You're at an exciting stage of change in which your commitment should be starting to translate into control. Enjoy the feeling of mastery that naturally results from managing your food to balance your energy equation. You've worked hard to develop your portion perception, and you should be proud.

Embrace your enthusiasm for a healthy new mind-set—but don't obsess. If you throw all your effort and energy into your eating plan, you may end up disappointed when it doesn't instantly solve your personal problems or land you a new job. Continue to nurture your relationships with yourself, other people, work, spirit, and all your life priorities.

Outside of your scheduled mealtimes, let go of thoughts about food. Everything you need to do is written down here, and you can consult it when it's time. So give your conscious mind a break, let your subconscious mind incubate the new skills you're learning, and attend to all the other important things in your life.

Living and eating well is easy once you have the right habits and mind-set. So take it easy on yourself.

FRIDAY, DAY 26

➤ Granola can be high in fat and calories. Buy a fat-free or low-fat brand and portion it carefully.

Breakfast	PS 1	PS 2	PS 3
Sweetened, nonfat yogurt	1 C.	1 C.	1 C.
Diced fresh fruit	½ C.	¾ C.	1 C.
Low-fat cereal (granola, Grape-Nuts, etc.)	½ oz.	1 oz.	1½ oz.
Calories	**300**	**375**	**450**

➤ The rice, beans, and tortillas featured in many Mexican dishes are healthy foods—but lard and full-fat sour cream and cheese are not!

Lunch			
Cooked beans (pinto, kidney, black, lentils, etc.)	½ C.	¾ C.	¾ C.
Cooked brown rice	⅓ C.	½ C.	¾ C.
Salsa	Unlimited	Unlimited	Unlimited
Low-fat tortilla	1 8-inch	1 10-inch	1 10-inch
Grated low-fat cheddar cheese	1 T.	1 T.	1 T.
Fat-free sour cream	1 T.	1 T.	1 T.
OR Vegetarian Burrito*	PS 1	PS 2	PS 3
Calories	**329**	**435**	**518**

➤ Get a bigger dose of good fish by swapping it for the chicken or pork at Monday's or Wednesday's dinner.

Dinner			
Fresh fish fillet	5 oz.	6 oz.	8 oz.
Any Portion Savvy Recipe sauce*	2 T.	2 T.	3 T.
OR Ginger-Crusted Salmon*	PS 1	PS 2	PS 3
Cooked rice or grains	½ C.	¾ C.	¾ C.
OR any Portion Savvy Recipe side dish*	PS 1	PS 2	PS 3
Steamed or grilled vegetables	1 C.	1½ C.	1½ C.
Calories	**356**	**456**	**529**

* See the Portion Savvy Recipes beginning on page 157.
For vegetarian alternatives, see page 209.

Friday Night with Friends and Family

Friday is a traditional night to gather with friends and family to share a meal. After a week of work and busy schedules, this is a time to celebrate your accomplishments, swap stories, and enjoy the natural recharge of being with people you love.

Tonight, make a special point of sharing your meal with the people who matter to you most. Cook up a delicious seafood dinner and portion it well, light some candles or cut some fresh flowers for a celebratory atmosphere, and experience the many levels at which the communal table can nurture and sustain you.

Portion Savvy Empowerment: Take Responsibility

Control is the goal of becoming portion savvy, and food is one of the few areas of your life that you can directly control every single day. That knowledge can make people feel even worse when they eat too much or indulge in something unintended. The message from your mind is, "You've lost control," which can lead to self-punishment and further overeating.

But I have a liberating truth: You *choose* your slipups. Every once in a while, it's natural to elect to relinquish control. If you've eaten something you regret, turn off your self-judgment and let it be. Don't beat yourself up. Realize that you decided to do what you did; you'll choose differently tomorrow, and that's just one day's delay in achieving benefits you'll enjoy your whole life. Your last meal is never as important as your next one.

Meanwhile, you've learned something about the internal or external triggers that can get between you and your goals. What are they? Write them down to set yourself free.

SATURDAY, DAY 27

➤ At juice bars, stick to fruit, soy beverage, and protein powder and order an 8- to 12-ounce small. This is a meal!

Breakfast	PS 1	PS 2	PS 3
Light vanilla soy beverage	1 c.	1½ c.	2 c.
Protein powder	2 T.	2 T.	2 T.
Fresh fruit	¾ c.	1 c.	1¼ c.
Calories	**295**	**380**	**465**

➤ Monitor the size *and* content of your burgers. Stick to poultry, seafood, or soy and skip the cheese, mayo, and dressing.

Lunch			
Ground turkey or chicken breast, salmon, lean beef, or soy burger mixture (raw) OR BBQ Chicken, Salmon, or Soy Burger*	4 oz.	6 oz.	8 oz.
Bun, bread, or English muffin	1½ oz.	2 oz.	2 oz.
Lettuce, tomato, onion, mustard, pickles	Unlimited	Unlimited	Unlimited
Fat-free mayonnaise, ketchup, relish	Up to 1 T.	Up to 1 T.	Up to 2 T.
Jicama Slaw*	½ c.	½ c.	½ c.
OR Cucumber Salad*	PS1	PS2	PS2
Calories	**345**	**450**	**510**

➤ On pizzas, emphasize the vegetables, take it easy on cheese, avoid fatty meats— and always plate your pizza serving before eating!

Dinner			
Medium 12" pizza	1 slice	2 slices	2½ slices
OR any Portion Savvy Recipe pizza*	2 slices	3 slices	4 slices
Mixed greens	Unlimited	Unlimited	Unlimited
Fat-free salad dressing	2 T.	2 T.	2 T.
Calories	**275**	**400**	**525**

* See the Portion Savvy Recipes beginning on page 157.

Downsize Your Dishes

Your right-size servings can look small on a huge dinner plate. Today, rearrange your cupboards to make your smallest plates, bowls, and glasses easily accessible. Move your big dinner plates to a far corner for long-term storage and use smaller sizes or salad plates for most meals. Extra-large tumblers are for water only, please! Try serving everything onto dishes one size smaller than you would normally choose. Watch your portions grow before your eyes!

Portion Savvy Empowerment: See Your Self-Confidence

Confidence is key to everything from success on the job to feeling good in social situations to sticking with your healthy habits. The trouble is that you can't always summon up confidence on demand. Here's a creative visualization that can help.

As you enter any intimidating situation, don't worry about looking at the other people there. Instead, focus on how they see you: poised, calm, attractive, smiling, charismatic. Now act like this person, playing the role as if you were in a movie. Watch your performance with pleasure. It's going just fine!

When you act as if you're self-confident, the world accepts you as such. Your mind is a great trickster, and just as it can give you the false message that you're not good enough, you can pretend not to hear. Your mischievous mind surrenders and lets your imagined scenario become reality. When you visualize self-confidence, the real thing soon comes along.

SUNDAY, DAY 28

	Breakfast	PS 1	PS 2	PS 3
➤ Don't skip breakfast! Not only does it refuel your brain and body after a long night of fasting, but it also kicks your fat-burning metabolism into gear.	Multi-Grain Pie*	1 piece	1 piece	1½ pieces
	Orange, grapefruit, or tomato juice	½ c.	¾ c.	1 c.
	Nonfat milk	1 c.	1 c.	1 c.
	Calories	**261**	**336**	**444**

	Lunch			
➤ Enjoy plenty of vegetarian meals for health, and solve potential protein problems by incorporating food pairs with complementary amino acids: dairy and grains, grains and legumes, or legumes and seeds.	Asparagus, Lima Bean, and Bow-Tie Pasta Salad* OR Tabbouleh and Tomato Pilaf*	1½ c.	2 c.	2½ c.
	Calories	**324**	**433**	**540**

	Dinner			
➤ When you indulge in red meat, use one of the leanest cuts and weigh it for your portion size. I recommend eating beef no more than twice a month; try the Turkey Stew for the intervening weeks.	Burgundy Beef Stew*	1½ c.	2 c.	2½ c.
	OR Turkey Stew*	2½ c.	3 c.	3½ c.
	Calories	**334**	**445**	**556**

* See the Portion Savvy Recipes beginning on page 157.

Portion Savvy Pleasures

The weekend is a wonderful time to enjoy life's many calorie-free pleasures. Building plenty of relaxation and fun into your day is the best way to keep yourself well nourished without overeating, but busy lives often threaten to preempt such natural rewards.

Here are some ways to treat yourself today. Copy them into your journal and add your favorites, then enjoy these activities as often as you can. This also makes a great "instead of" list; whenever you're tempted to nibble outside of your eating plan, turn to your list and have one of these healthy pleasures instead.

➤ Read a novel, a biography of someone you admire, or a frivolous magazine you don't usually grant yourself the time for.
➤ Paint or draw.
➤ Read or write poetry.
➤ Dig through your music collection for an old favorite you haven't heard for a long time.
➤ Get outside and enjoy nature.
➤ Play a game, maybe with your mate or children.
➤ Rent a funny movie and laugh a lot.

Portion Savvy Empowerment: Practice Patience

Occasionally you do everything right but the results don't follow. In weight loss, we call this a plateau—when you're eating less than you're expending, but your body doesn't seem to change.

First, realize that your body can send out all kinds of false signals—retaining water, replacing fat with heavier muscle mass, shrinking in a place that you didn't think to check. Second, understand that plateaus are a natural part of physiological change. Emptying out fat stores, building muscles, and redesigning your metabolism has inherent ebbs and flows, so go with it, just as if you were floating down a river. Tell yourself, "My body just hasn't caught up with my expectations." Continue with your good habits, don't try to rush or force, have faith, and the pounds will inevitably surrender.

GRADUATION: CALM
LAUNCH YOUR NEW LIFE

The final two days of the Portion Savvy 30-Day Plan review what you've learned during the past four weeks and provide an action plan for taking your new, healthy habits into the future. This is your graduation! In fact, the transition from *learning how* to *being* portion savvy is not unlike college commencement, in which your mentors offer well-earned congratulations, then deliver the news that you have the knowledge, the structure, and the discipline you need—now go get a job.

Your job is to keep on doing what you now know how to do. These two days will help you move from following my detailed instructions to planning for yourself. As you move out on your own, you'll experience the deep **calm** that personal control brings. Balanced and serene, you know everything you need to be your best.

Graduation and Beyond!—Game Plan

➤ Assess your progress. Take this time to evaluate your PS level. Has your weight loss so far bumped you down to a lower level? Check the chart on page 32 to find out and adjust your portions accordingly. Remember that when you're ready to move from weight loss to maintenance mode, all you need to do is adopt the PS level one higher than your last level for weight loss. (If, after two weeks at your new maintenance level, you find you've gained weight, adjust by cutting out a snack each day; if you've lost weight, add a daily snack. If the disequilibrium continues for two more weeks, move one PS level.)

➤ Recalculate your BMI to measure your progress toward your goal in the Fit range.

➤ Use the meal plans from Weeks One to Four as examples to help you plan your future menus as explained in Day 29. Don't forget your designated snacks!

➤ Stick with the Week Four workout program. Exercise is an integral element of your portion savvy habits and is as important for maintenance as it is for burning fat. Keep a move on!

➤ Continue to make entries in your food journal and scrapbook until you reach your goal. After that, it's up to you. Jot down a thought, make a sketch, or paste in a photo whenever you like. Refer to these pages frequently to refresh your memory, boost your motivation, or congratulate yourself on your progress.

ASSESS YOUR PROGRESS

Refer to the instructions on pages 30, 33, and 59 for the self-assessments below. Recalculating your BMR will allow you to adjust your PS level if necessary. Check your metabolic rate once a month during weight loss to keep your energy equation accurate!

Weight_____   BMR_____   BMI_____

Measurements

Chest (at widest point)   _____

Bicep (at widest point)   _____

Waist ($\frac{1}{2}$" above belly button)   _____

Hips (stand with feet together and
    measure at widest point of buttocks)   _____

Right thigh (just below buttocks)   _____

Clothes fit test (check any that are looser or fill in your new size):

_____ Pants _____ Skirt _____ Shirt or blouse _____ Blazer or jacket

Present weight goal range _____

MONDAY, DAY 29: MAKE A SMART PLAN

You've got the skills, so from now on, *you* decide what you're going to eat. If a bagel is your favorite breakfast, have it as often as you like. Maybe you've fallen in love with the Veggie Burrito; schedule it a few times this week. Try salmon on Monday and stew on Tuesday. Every meal you've eaten on the Portion Savvy 30-Day Plan serves as a prototype for your portions; now you can mix and match them as you like. Variety is the spice of life—and also a nutritionally and psychologically sound way to eat!

All I ask is that you (1) plan in advance and (2) write it down. Planning not only helps you shop and cook calmly and efficiently, but it also helps preset your portions and keep you in the driver's seat. The margin for error on a planned menu is narrow, but improvisation invites mistakes.

Make many photocopies of the following form and sit down every week to fill in seven days of menus, including restaurant meals, takeout, and social occasions. Start today by planning the rest of your week, using for guidance the meals summarized in Week Four and the Portion Savvy Recipes. Lunch and dinner are interchangeable, so feel free to swap them to meet your tastes and needs.

This is the creative part. Have fun!

PS 1

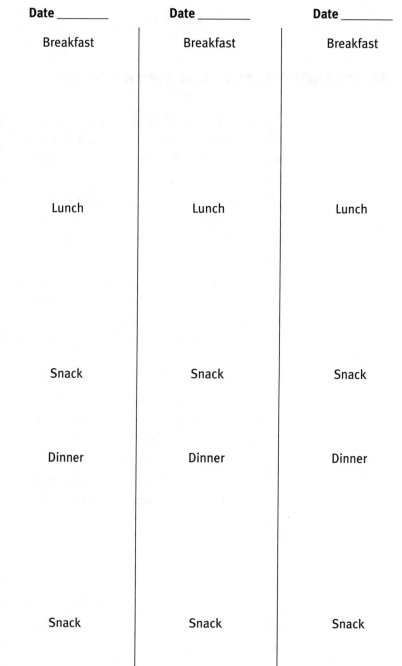

Date _____	Date _____	Date _____
Breakfast	Breakfast	Breakfast
Lunch	Lunch	Lunch
Snack	Snack	Snack
Dinner	Dinner	Dinner
Snack	Snack	Snack

PS 2

Date _____

Breakfast

Snack

Lunch

Snack

Dinner

Snack

Date _____

Breakfast

Snack

Lunch

Snack

Dinner

Snack

Date _____

Breakfast

Snack

Lunch

Snack

Dinner

Snack

PS 3

Date _____	Date _____	Date _____
Breakfast	Breakfast	Breakfast
Snack	Snack	Snack
Lunch	Lunch	Lunch
Snack	Snack	Snack
Snack	Snack	Snack
Dinner	Dinner	Dinner
Snack	Snack	Snack

Portion Savvy Empowerment: Success Is in the Details

You've probably realized that a big part of being portion savvy is keeping track of the details of your eating life, the same way that you keep your checkbook balanced, the laundry done, and the car maintained. Like any good manager, you set yourself some rules and timetables, follow them—and then enjoy the resulting success.

At Diet Designs, each client receives a weekly meal plan with every meal and snack spelled out. I work closely with people to help them plan their weekends, social events, and restaurant meals all around the world. My clients have proven my motto that there's no portion problem you can't solve with a plan.

At the National Weight Control Registry, 60 percent of the successful dieters got strict with themselves. Many planned their meals a week in advance, and detailed food journals were a favorite control strategy.

Make a smart plan to keep your meals, snacks, and exercise sessions under control. When you manage the details, the big picture takes care of itself.

TUESDAY, DAY 30: REVIEW

Today, your last day of training, I'd like you to take some time to review the skills you've learned and the tools at your disposal. Everyone who's ever taken a final exam knows that review is the key to imprinting facts and concepts into your memory so that you can recall them even under the duress of a hushed examination room or noisy restaurant.

Meanwhile, follow the meal plan you created yesterday. Fill in any holes that might be left so that you can start tomorrow, your first day as a portion savvy graduate, with everything in place for success.

So if this is the review, you ask, what's the test?

It sounds dramatic, but every client I've set free to fly knows it's true: The test is the rest of your life.

Test Your Tools

Get out all the following measurement tools and assemble them on a table or countertop:

- ➤ Portion savvy pop-outs
- ➤ Kitchen scale
- ➤ Dry measuring cups
- ➤ Liquid measuring cups
- ➤ Measuring spoons
- ➤ Your designated cereal bowl
- ➤ Your designated juice glass

Now, test yourself. For each tool in turn, try to remember all the foods on the Portion Savvy Plan that can be measured with it. Check your answers with the correct ones in the box.

Answers
- ➤ Portion savvy pop-outs: fruit, muffins, poultry and meat, seafood, cooked rice or grains, potatoes.
- ➤ Scale: cereal, bagels, muffins, bread, rolls, dry pasta, poultry, seafood, meat, burgers, cheese, potatoes.
- ➤ Dry measuring cups: chopped fruit and vegetables, cottage cheese, yogurt, cooked pasta, cooked rice and grains, cooked beans, pasta salad.
- ➤ Liquid measuring cups: juice, milk, soy beverage, egg substitute, tomato sauce, soup, stew.
- ➤ Measuring spoons: cream cheese, cottage cheese, fruit preserves, protein powder, grated cheese, salad dressing, nonfat sour cream, sauce.
- ➤ Bowl: cereal.
- ➤ Glass: juice.

Study Up

You can use your measurement tools to prepare to take your portion perception on the road. Part of being portion savvy is making good decisions that keep your energy equation balanced anytime, anywhere. When you're far from your portion-controlled kitchen, a little studying can go a long way.

Before any meal out, decide what you'll order or, for a meal at someone else's home, inquire about the menu if possible. Write down what you plan to eat, including your PS serving sizes.

Now take out the portion savvy pop-outs or appropriate measuring tools for those items. Pick each one up individually and look at it carefully, memorizing the outline so you can picture your serving on the plate later on. Review your scrapbook for photographs of any relevant portions. Study them until your portion perception clicks in.

Savvy Shopping

You've spent four weeks making your kitchen a portion savvy place, but you can start smart at the supermarket to put the portioning process in gear before your food even comes through your front door. The tips below work with your weekly meal plans to add the final touch of grace to your new habits.

➤ Use your meal plan to make a shopping list organized by store section. Start by visualizing your supermarket and planning your route so that your last three stops are the produce, meat and seafood, and freezer sections, respectively. Write your list to follow your route.

➤ Develop a weekly marketing schedule:
  • Stock up anytime on nonperishable items such as canned beans and soups, defatted low-sodium broth, pasta, grains, marinara sauce, condiments, salad dressing, snacks, and frozen juice.
  • Buy fresh foods regularly on a schedule that fits your household's needs. Pick up fresh fruit, vegetables, poultry, seafood, meat, dairy products, and bread on these stops. Don't overbuy fresh foods, though extra is okay if it freezes well.

➤ Bring along your portion savvy pop-outs for quick size checks.

➤ Buy the smallest available size of everything. Look for individual packages—small boxes of raisins, 8-ounce cartons of yogurt, and so forth.

➤ Use the scale in the produce department to size potatoes.

➤ Have your poultry, seafood, meat, and deli items cut to your serving size. Full-service counters will cut anything to order; if your supermarket doesn't offer this service, consider switching to one that does.

➤ Portion food immediately when you get home, wrapping up individual servings and refrigerating or freezing if necessary.

Portion Savvy Empowerment: Living Better from Within

Living better begins when we establish order within so that order can become a visible reality in our lives every day.

Be still. Be present in the moment. Be aware of everything within you and everything around you.

Today, tomorrow, and every day that follows, let the balance, focus, and direction you hold inside make itself manifest in your beautiful body and self-loving behavior. It's as natural as breathing.

PART III

PORTION SAVVY RECIPES

Breakfast
Apple-Raisin Bran Muffins
Cherry–Oat Bran Muffins
Chive Spread
Fruit Spread
Multi-Grain Pie

Lunch
Asparagus, Lima Bean, and Bow-Tie Pasta Salad
Barbecue Chicken Burger
Minestrone
Pasta with Lentil Sauce
Salmon Burger
Southwestern Chicken Salad
Soy Burger
Tabbouleh and Tomato Pilaf
Vegetarian Burrito

Dinner
Burgundy Beef Stew
Ginger-Crusted Salmon
Greek Feta Chicken
Pizza Crust
Pizza with Chicken and Broccoli
Pizza with Fennel and Pine Nuts
Pizza with Shrimp, Mushrooms, and Red Pepper
Polenta Lasagna
Pork Marbella
Turkey Stew
Turkey Tetrazzini

Sides and Salads
Butternut Squash Purée
Creamed Spinach
Cucumber Salad

Jicama Slaw
Mustard Potatoes
Orange Couscous
Papaya Rice
Roasted Root Vegetables
Wild Rice Pilaf

**Sauces,
Rubs, and
Dressings**

Artichoke Pesto
Herb Vinaigrette
Honey-Chili Sauce
House Marinara
Lemon-Cumin Rub
Lime-Soy Vinaigrette
Marbella Sauce
Mustard Cream Sauce
Papaya Marinade
Papaya Vinaigrette
Port Wine Sauce
Raspberry Vinaigrette
Rosemary Rub
Salsa Fresca
Yogurt Sauce

Desserts

Apple Cobbler
Caramel Bars
Chocolate-Orange Biscotti
Date Purée
Molasses Cookies
Oatmeal Chocolate Chip Cookies
White Chocolate Meringue Drops

BREAKFAST

APPLE-RAISIN BRAN MUFFINS

PS LEVEL	SERVING	CALORIES	% FROM FAT	FAT	PROTEIN	CARB.	CHOL.	SODIUM
PS 1–3	1 muffin	247	3.2%	1.0 g	6.3 g	60.3 g	1 mg	208 mg

These moist, satisfying muffins provide both soluble fiber in the apples and insoluble fiber in the wheat bran.

1 pound seedless raisins

1 cup water

2 cups wheat bran

½ cup low-fat buttermilk

½ cup frozen apple juice concentrate, thawed

½ cup sugar

1 cup all-purpose flour

1 teaspoon baking powder

1 teaspoon baking soda

1 tablespoon ground cinnamon

Dash salt

1 large apple, grated

7 egg whites

½ teaspoon vanilla extract

1. Combine the raisins and the water in a microwave-safe dish, cover, and cook on high for 5 minutes or until raisins are soft. Drain excess liquid and purée the raisins in a food processor until smooth.

2. In a large mixing bowl, combine the bran, buttermilk, apple juice concentrate, and sugar. Add the raisin purée and stir well to combine. Let mixture stand for 20 minutes. (Or cover and refrigerate overnight; return to room temperature before proceeding.)

3. Preheat the oven to 350 degrees. Line a twelve-cup muffin tin with paper muffin cups and mist lightly with cooking spray.

4. In another bowl, sift together the flour, baking powder, soda, cinnamon, and salt.

5. Grate the apple in a food processor. Add the egg whites and vanilla to the bran mixture and stir to combine. Stir in the flour mixture, then the grated apple.

6. Spoon ½ cup of batter into each prepared muffin cup and bake until crusty on top, about 20–30 minutes.

Yields twelve 3-ounce muffins.

CHERRY-OAT BRAN MUFFINS

PS LEVEL	SERVING	CALORIES	% FROM FAT	FAT	PROTEIN	CARB.	CHOL.	SODIUM
PS 1–3	1 muffin	238	3.0%	0.9 g	5.5 g	56.2 g	0 mg	276 mg

Dried cherries add a different touch to your morning starter.

2¼ cups all-purpose flour

¾ cup oat bran

¾ cup firmly packed light brown sugar

4 teaspoons baking powder

½ teaspoon salt

2 teaspoons ground cinnamon

¾ cup Date Purée (see recipe on page 206)

¾ cup skim milk

⅓ cup maple syrup

3 egg whites, lightly beaten with a fork

1⅓ cups chopped frozen and thawed pitted cherries

⅓ cup dried cherries

1. Preheat the oven to 375 degrees. Line a twelve-cup muffin tin with paper muffin cups and mist lightly with cooking spray.

2. In a large mixing bowl, combine the flour, oat bran, brown sugar, baking powder, salt, and cinnamon. Stir to combine.

3. In a separate bowl, beat together the Date Purée, milk, maple syrup, egg whites, and frozen and dried cherries.

4. Add the wet to the dry ingredients and stir just until moistened.

5. Spoon ½ cup batter into each prepared muffin cup and bake 25–30 minutes, or until lightly browned.

Yields twelve 3-ounce muffins.

CHIVE SPREAD

PS LEVEL	SERVING	CALORIES	% FROM FAT	FAT	PROTEIN	CARB.	CHOL.	SODIUM
PS 1	2 T.	35	0.0%	0.0 g	5.0 g	2.0 g	6 mg	186 mg
PS 2 & 3	3 T.	53	0.0%	0.0 g	7.5 g	3.0 g	9 mg	279 mg

Make a batch of Chive or Fruit Spread to spread on your bagels all week!

1 cup fat-free cream cheese, softened
4 teaspoons minced chives
2 teaspoons minced capers

1. In a small bowl, cream together the cream cheese, chives, and capers with an electric mixer until smooth. Chill until ready to serve.
2. Serve with bagels.
Yields 1 cup.

FRUIT SPREAD

PS LEVEL	SERVING	CALORIES	% FROM FAT	FAT	PROTEIN	CARB.	CHOL.	SODIUM
PS 1	2 T.	53	0.0%	0.0 g	5.0 g	8.4 g	6 mg	184 mg
PS 2 & 3	3 T.	79	0.0%	0.0 g	7.5 g	12.6 g	9 mg	276 mg

1 cup fat-free cream cheese, softened
¼ cup fruit-sweetened preserves

1. In a small bowl, cream together the cream cheese and preserves with an electric mixer until smooth. Chill until ready to serve.
2. Serve with bagels.
Yields 1 cup.

MULTI-GRAIN PIE

PS LEVEL	SERVING	CALORIES	% FROM FAT	FAT	PROTEIN	CARB.	CHOL.	SODIUM
PS 1 & 2	1 piece	156	5.1%	0.9 g	3.6 g	35.0 g	0 mg	125 mg
PS 3	1½ pieces	234	5.1%	1.4 g	5.4 g	52.5 g	0 mg	188 mg

A cross between hot cereal and a casserole, Multi-Grain Pie sticks to your ribs but not to your fat cells.

⅜ cup steel-cut oats
⅜ cup raw brown rice
⅜ cup raw pearl barley
⅜ cup raw bulgur
⅜ cup diced apricots (about 8 halves)
⅜ cup diced pitted dates (about 6 dates)
½ cup plus 2 tablespoons dark brown sugar, divided
½ teaspoon salt
4 cups water
2 teaspoons ground cinnamon

1. Preheat the oven to 350 degrees. Coat a 9-by-9-inch baking dish with cooking spray.

2. In a large bowl, combine the oats, rice, barley, bulgur, apricots, dates, ½ cup dark brown sugar, salt, and water. Mix well.

3. Transfer the grain mixture to the baking dish. Cover loosely with foil and bake, stirring occasionally, until water is absorbed, grains are tender, and mixture is creamy, about 45 minutes. Meanwhile, combine the remaining 2 tablespoons dark brown sugar with the cinnamon in a small bowl.

4. Uncover the casserole, sprinkle with the brown sugar and cinnamon, and bake for 10 to 15 minutes more to brown the top. Cool on a wire rack before cutting.

Yields 9 pieces.

TO PORTION: Cut into 9 pieces, 3 each way.

LUNCH

Lunches and dinners are interchangeable on the Portion Savvy Plan.

ASPARAGUS, LIMA BEAN, AND BOW-TIE PASTA SALAD

PS LEVEL	SERVING	CALORIES	% FROM FAT	FAT	PROTEIN	CARB.	CHOL.	SODIUM
PS 1	1½ cups	324	14.7%	5.3 g	12.3 g	57.4 g	1 mg	246 mg
PS 2	2 cups	433	14.7%	7.1 g	16.4 g	76.5 g	1 mg	328 mg
PS 3	2½ cups	540	14.7%	9.0 g	20.5 g	95.8 g	2 mg	410 mg

Use the leftover Artichoke Pesto to top pasta, chicken, or seafood later in the week.

Artichoke Pesto
8 ounces canned artichoke hearts, drained and coarsely chopped
2 tablespoons toasted pine nuts
2 tablespoons grated Parmesan cheese
2 tablespoons chopped fresh basil
2 teaspoons chopped fresh parsley
2 teaspoons chopped garlic
¼ cup dry white wine
2 tablespoons fresh lemon juice
2 tablespoons fat-free, reduced-sodium chicken or vegetable broth
Dash each salt, black pepper, and cayenne pepper

1 tablespoon olive oil
¾ cup chopped onion
2 teaspoons minced garlic
¼ cup thinly sliced reconstituted sun-dried tomatoes (packed without oil)
½ pound asparagus, cut on the diagonal
¾ cup frozen baby lima beans
8 ounces farfalle (bow-tie) pasta
Salt and freshly ground black pepper

1. Prepare the Artichoke Pesto by combining all the ingredients in a food processor or blender and puréeing until smooth. Set aside ½ cup sauce and freeze the rest in ½-cup portions for use in this recipe or in your PS serving to top chicken or fish.

2. Set a large pot of water to boil.

3. Heat the oil in a skillet over medium heat. Add the onion, garlic, and tomatoes and sauté until tender, about 5 minutes. Set aside.

4. Blanch the asparagus in the boiling water until just tender, about 3–5 minutes. Scoop out, drain, and refresh with cold water.

5. Add the lima beans and pasta to the boiling water and cook until both are tender, about 8 minutes. Drain.

6. Toss the pasta and beans with the asparagus, tomato mixture, ½ cup Artichoke Pesto, and salt and pepper. Serve hot or cold.

Yields 6 cups.

BARBECUE CHICKEN BURGER

PS LEVEL	SERVING	CALORIES	% FROM FAT	FAT	PROTEIN	CARB.	CHOL.	SODIUM
PS 1	4 oz. with 1½-oz. bun	228	11.0%	2.7 g	18.3 g	32.1 g	31 mg	578 mg
PS 2	6 oz. with 2-oz. bun	327	11.0%	4.0 g	26.8 g	45.3 g	46 mg	831 mg
PS 3	8 oz. with 2-oz. bun	391	11.1%	4.8 g	34.1 g	51.8 g	61 mg	999 mg

Barbecue sauce keeps these patties moist; you won't miss the beef!

2 tablespoons fat-free, reduced-sodium chicken broth
¾ cup diced onions
1 teaspoon minced garlic
14 ounces ground chicken breast meat
½ cup barbecue sauce
1 tablespoon Worcestershire sauce
1 teaspoon Dijon mustard
1 teaspoon ground thyme
¾ cup fresh bread crumbs
Hamburger buns

1. Heat the chicken broth in a small skillet over medium heat. Add the onions and sauté until caramelized, 5 to 10 minutes. Add the garlic and cook for 5 minutes more. Set aside to cool.

2. In a mixing bowl, combine the onion mixture with all the remaining ingredients except buns. Stir well. Form into six 4-ounce patties for PS 1, four 6-ounce patties for PS 2, or three 8-ounce patties for PS 3.

3. Coat a nonstick skillet with cooking spray, place over medium heat, and cook burgers until no longer pink—about 4 minutes per side for 4-ounce patties, 5 minutes per side for 6-ounce patties, and 6 minutes per side for 8-ounce patties.

4. Serve with a bun according to your PS level and fat-free condiments of choice.

VARIATION: Substitute ground turkey breast for the chicken.
Yields 24 ounces.

MINESTRONE

PS LEVEL	SERVING	CALORIES	% FROM FAT	FAT	PROTEIN	CARB.	CHOL.	SODIUM
PS 1–3	2 c.	191	3.6%	1.0 g	23.6 g	35.3 g	0 mg	386 mg

Make a pot of soup over the weekend to cover several weekday lunches; the flavors blend as it sits.

7¼ cups fat-free, reduced-sodium chicken broth, divided

1 onion, chopped

1 tablespoon chopped garlic

1 cup diced celery

1 cup diced carrots

4 cups low-fat marinara sauce (bottled, or see the House Marinara recipe on page 197)

3 Roma tomatoes, peeled, seeded, and chopped

1 bay leaf

1 cup cooked white beans (drained and rinsed if canned)

3 ounces raw orzo pasta

3 ounces fresh spinach

2 tablespoons fresh basil, chopped

2 tablespoons fresh oregano, chopped

1 teaspoon balsamic vinegar

Freshly ground black pepper

1. Heat ¼ cup chicken broth in a soup pot over medium heat. Add the onions and garlic and sauté until translucent, 5 to 10 minutes.

2. Add the celery, carrots, marinara sauce, tomatoes, bay leaf, and remaining 7 cups chicken broth. Simmer, partially covered, for 20 minutes.

3. Add the beans, orzo, spinach, basil, oregano, vinegar, and freshly ground black pepper to taste. Return to a simmer, cook for 15 minutes more, and serve.

Yields 12 cups.

PASTA WITH LENTIL SAUCE

PS LEVEL	SERVING	CALORIES	% FROM FAT	FAT	PROTEIN	CARB.	CHOL.	SODIUM
PS 1	1 c. pasta with ³/₄ c. sauce	322	4.8%	1.7 g	17.4 g	63.5 g	0 mg	283 mg
PS 2	1¹/₂ c. pasta with 1 c. sauce	463	4.7%	2.4 g	24.3 g	91.5 g	0 mg	377 mg
PS 3	1³/₄ c. pasta with 1¹/₄ c. sauce	554	4.7%	2.9 g	29.5 g	109.3 g	0 mg	471 mg

This hearty combination will satisfy your deepest carbohydrate cravings.

¹/₂ cup plus 2 tablespoons fat-free, reduced-sodium chicken broth, divided

¹/₂ cup chopped onion

¹/₂ cup chopped carrot

2 teaspoons minced garlic

³/₈ cup dried lentils

1¹/₂ cups canned chopped tomatoes, undrained

1¹/₂ teaspoons sugar

¹/₂ teaspoon ground cumin

¹/₂ teaspoon ground ginger

¹/₂ teaspoon dried basil

¹/₄ teaspoon paprika

¹/₈ teaspoon cayenne pepper

6 ounces corkscrew pasta

6 ounces fresh spinach, well washed, dried, chopped

¼ cup plain, nonfat yogurt

1. Heat 2 tablespoons chicken broth in a medium saucepan over medium heat. Add the onion, carrot, and garlic and sauté for 5 minutes, adding more stock if the mixture dries out.

2. Add the remaining broth and the lentils, tomatoes, sugar, cumin, ginger, basil, paprika, and cayenne. Bring to a simmer and cook, partially covered, for 30 minutes or until the lentils are tender.

3. Meanwhile, bring a large pot of water to a boil and cook the pasta according to package directions.

4. Remove the lentil sauce from the heat and stir in the spinach until wilted. Add the yogurt and combine well. Toss the sauce and hot pasta as called for by your PS level together and serve.

Yields 3 cups pasta and 3 cups sauce.

SALMON BURGER

PS LEVEL	SERVING	CALORIES	% FROM FAT	FAT	PROTEIN	CARB.	CHOL.	SODIUM
PS 1	4 oz. with 1½-oz. bun	235	16.6%	4.3 g	21.1 g	27.5 g	39 mg	389 mg
PS 2	6 oz. with 2-oz. bun	336	17.0%	6.3 g	31.0 g	38.1 g	59 mg	543 mg
PS 3	8 oz. with 2-oz. bun	403	18.0%	8.0 g	39.6 g	42.2 g	79 mg	615 mg

This really is a betterburger: packed with omega-3 oils to keep your arteries clear!

½ cup fresh bread crumbs

2 egg whites

½ cup chopped green onions

1 tablespoon chopped fresh dill weed

1 tablespoon chopped capers

3 tablespoons fresh lemon juice

1 teaspoon paprika

¼ teaspoon dry mustard

¼ teaspoon black pepper

Dash cayenne pepper

1 pound salmon fillet
Hamburger buns

1. Preheat the oven to 350 degrees. In a mixing bowl, combine the bread crumbs, egg whites, green onion, dill, capers, lemon juice, paprika, mustard, pepper, and cayenne. Stir to combine well.

2. Grind the salmon with gentle pulses in the food processor or with the grinder attachment of a KitchenAid mixer. Add the salmon to the bread crumb mixture and mix gently just until combined.

3. Form into six 4-ounce patties for PS 1, four 6-ounce patties for PS 2, or three 8-ounce patties for PS 3.

4. Coat a baking sheet with cooking spray. Arrange the burgers on the pan and bake until just cooked through, about 4 minutes total for 4-ounce patties, 6 minutes for 6-ounce patties, and 8 minutes for 8-ounce patties.

5. Serve with a bun according to your PS level and fat-free condiments of choice.

Yields 24 ounces.

SOUTHWESTERN CHICKEN SALAD

PS LEVEL	SERVING	CALORIES	% FROM FAT	FAT	PROTEIN	CARB.	CHOL.	SODIUM
PS 1 & 2	1 salad with 4 oz. chicken	271	7.8%	2.5 g	25.3 g	40.6 g	53 mg	113 mg
PS 3	1 salad with 6 oz. chicken	321	8.2%	3.1 g	35.8 g	40.6 g	79 mg	142 mg

Try this sweet and savory marinade with any grilled chicken, fish, or pork tenderloin.

Papaya Marinade

1 cup papaya nectar
3 tablespoons fresh orange juice
3 tablespoons fresh lemon juice
½ teaspoon minced garlic
½ teaspoon ground cinnamon
½ teaspoon ground cumin
1 teaspoon brown sugar
2 teaspoons honey mustard

1 teaspoon chili sauce

2 dashes liquid-smoke flavoring

1 pound (PS 1 and 2) or 1½ pounds (PS 3) boneless, skinless chicken
    breasts

1 medium red onion, sliced

1 medium mango, peeled, seeded, and sliced

1 medium jicama, peeled and sliced

1 pound mixed baby greens

2 oranges, peeled and sectioned

½ cup canned corn, drained

1. To make the Papaya Marinade, combine all the ingredients in a food processor or blender and process until combined.

2. Place the chicken breasts in a nonreactive dish and pour ¾ cup of marinade over them. Let marinate for 1 hour at room temperature or up to overnight covered in the refrigerator.

3. Meanwhile, reserve ½ cup of the remaining marinade and set aside. Place the onion, mango, and jicama in a nonreactive dish and pour the unreserved marinade over them.

4. Preheat the grill or broiler. Remove the chicken, onion, and mango from the marinade and grill or broil on both sides until cooked through. Cut the chicken breasts into lengthwise strips and separate the onion into rings.

5. To assemble the salads, divide the baby greens evenly among four plates. Top with one quarter each of the chicken strips, the jicama, grilled red onion rings, orange sections, and 2 tablespoons corn kernels. Top with the grilled mango, then sprinkle each salad with 2 tablespoons of the reserved marinade.

Serves 4.

SOY BURGER

PS LEVEL	SERVING	CALORIES	% FROM FAT	FAT	PROTEIN	CARB.	CHOL.	SODIUM
PS 1	4 oz. with 1½-oz. bun	259	16.9%	5.0 g	12.4 g	42.6 g	30 mg	449 mg
PS 2	6 oz. with 2-oz. bun	372	17.3%	7.3 g	17.9 g	60.7 g	45 mg	633 mg
PS 3	8 oz. with 2-oz. bun	451	18.1%	9.3 g	22.2 g	72.4 g	60 mg	735 mg

Superfood in a bun.

¾ cup finely chopped onion
¾ cup finely chopped carrot
¼ cup finely chopped red bell pepper
4 cloves garlic, minced
1 cup canned soybeans, drained, rinsed, and coarsely puréed
1¼ cups cooked basmati rice (may substitute long-grain white rice)
⅓ cup seasoned dry bread crumbs
3 tablespoons finely chopped fresh parsley
Tabasco sauce to taste
Salt and pepper to taste
1 egg
Hamburger buns

1. Preheat the oven to 350 degrees. Coat a medium, nonstick skillet with cooking spray and place over medium-high heat until hot. Add the onion, carrot, bell pepper, and garlic and sauté until tender, about 8 minutes.

2. Transfer the onion mixture to a mixing bowl and add the soybeans, rice, bread crumbs, and parsley. Mix to combine. Season to taste with Tabasco sauce, salt, and pepper. Add the egg and blend well.

3. Form the mixture into six 4-ounce patties for PS 1, four 6-ounce patties for PS 2, or three 8-ounce patties for PS 3.

4. Coat a baking sheet with cooking spray. Arrange the burgers on the pan and bake until cooked through, about 8 minutes total for 4-ounce patties, 9 minutes for 6-ounce patties, and 10 minutes for 8-ounce patties.

5. Serve with a bun according to your PS level and fat-free condiments of choice.

Yields 24 ounces.

TABBOULEH AND TOMATO PILAF

PS LEVEL	SERVING	CALORIES	% FROM FAT	FAT	PROTEIN	CARB.	CHOL.	SODIUM
PS 1	1½ cups pilaf with ¼ cup sauce	302	21.2%	7.1 g	12.7 g	51.6 g	2 mg	644 mg
PS 2	2 cups pilaf with ⅓ cup sauce	403	21.0%	9.4 g	16.9 g	68.8 g	3 mg	857 mg
PS 3	2½ cups with 6 T. sauce	503	21.1%	11.8 g	21.3 g	86.0 g	3 mg	1,069 mg

A cool echo of the Middle East.

1 cup raw tabbouleh
2 cups boiling water

Yogurt Sauce
¾ cup plain, nonfat yogurt
2 tablespoons nonfat sour cream
¼ cup fresh lime juice
1 tablespoon chopped parsley
1 tablespoon fresh dill
¼ teaspoon granulated garlic
Dash salt

2 cups canned garbanzo beans, drained and rinsed
1 cup diced plum tomatoes
1 cup chopped scallions
½ cup chopped parsley
1½ teaspoons grated lemon zest

¼ cup fresh lemon juice

½ teaspoon black pepper

1. Combine the tabbouleh and the water in a large bowl. Cover and let stand for 30 minutes.

2. Meanwhile, make the Yogurt Sauce: Combine the yogurt, sour cream, lime juice, parsley, dill, garlic, and salt and whisk until smooth. Cover and chill until ready to serve.

3. Add the garbanzo beans, tomatoes, scallions, parsley, lemon zest, lemon juice, and pepper to the tabbouleh. Combine well. Cover and chill until ready to serve.

4. Serve the pilaf topped with the Yogurt Sauce.

Yields 6 cups pilaf and 1 cup sauce.

VEGETARIAN BURRITO

PS LEVEL	SERVING	CALORIES	% FROM FAT	FAT	PROTEIN	CARB.	CHOL.	SODIUM
PS 1	1 c. filling with 8" tortilla	329	5.5%	2.0 g	15.0 g	63.1 g	3 mg	494 mg
PS 2	1⅓ c. filling with 10" tortilla	435	6.0%	2.9 g	19.6 g	85.4 g	4 mg	665 mg
PS 3	1¾ c. filling with 10" tortilla	518	5.7%	3.3 g	24.2 g	100.0 g	5 mg	730 mg

This Diet Designs classic was a client favorite long before the wrap craze.

1 cup dried pinto beans

1 cup raw brown rice

Salsa Fresca

1¼ cups chopped Roma tomatoes

¼ red onion, chopped

1 tablespoon chopped fresh cilantro

1 tablespoon fresh lime juice

¼ teaspoon minced serrano chili pepper

¼ cup fat-free, reduced-sodium chicken broth

½ teaspoon minced garlic

½ teaspoon chili powder

½ teaspoon ground cumin

½ cup diced carrots

¼ cup sliced scallions

2 tablespoons chopped fresh cilantro

4 tablespoons shredded, fat-free cheddar cheese

Salt to taste

Low-fat flour tortillas (five 8-inch for PS 1, four 10-inch for PS 2, three 10-inch for PS 3)

Fat-free sour cream (5 tablespoons for PS 1, 4 tablespoons for PS 2, 3 tablespoons for PS 3)

1. Cook the beans and the rice separately (see instructions on page 97). Drain.

2. Meanwhile, combine the ingredients for the Salsa Fresca and set aside.

3. Place the chicken broth in a small, nonstick skillet over medium heat. Add the garlic, chili powder, and cumin and sauté until the garlic is tender.

4. In a large bowl, combine the cooked rice and beans, the Salsa Fresca, the spice mixture, and the carrots, scallions, cilantro, cheddar cheese, and salt to taste.

5. Heat the tortillas for 30 seconds under the broiler or wrapped in plastic in the microwave. Portion the filling into the tortillas—1 cup into an 8-inch tortilla for PS 1, 1⅓ cups into a 10-inch tortilla for PS 2, and 1¾ cups into a 10-inch tortilla for PS 3—and roll up. Garnish each burrito with 1 tablespoon sour cream and serve.

Yields 5½ cups filling.

DINNER

Dinners and lunches are interchangeable on the Portion Savvy Plan.

BURGUNDY BEEF STEW

PS LEVEL	SERVING	CALORIES	% FROM FAT	FAT	PROTEIN	CARB.	CHOL.	SODIUM
PS 1	1½ c.	334	14.4%	4.9 g	33.5 g	31.5 g	82 mg	445 mg
PS 2	2 c.	445	14.4%	6.5 g	44.7 g	42.0 g	109 mg	593 mg
PS 3	2½ c.	556	14.4%	8.1 g	55.9 g	52.5 g	136 mg	741 mg

A delicious indulgence for your meat lover's soul.

8 ounces turkey bacon, diced

3 pounds lean beef tenderloin, cubed (may substitute chicken or turkey breast)

1 cup chopped onion

3 tablespoons flour

Salt and pepper to taste

5 cups diced red potatoes

3 cups Burgundy wine

3 cups defatted, low-sodium beef broth

2 tablespoons tomato paste

1 tablespoon chopped fresh rosemary

4 carrots, peeled and julienned

2 cups white pearl onions, peeled

1 tablespoon olive oil

8 ounces chanterelle mushrooms, sliced (may substitute other wild or domestic mushrooms)

1 tablespoon red currant jelly

2 tablespoons chopped Italian parsley

1. Preheat the oven to 300 degrees.

2. In a flameproof casserole dish, sauté the bacon over medium heat until crisp. Remove the bacon with a slotted spoon and discard, reserving the drippings.

3. Add the beef to the pan and sauté, stirring, until browned on all sides.

4. Add the chopped onions to the pan, then sprinkle with the flour and salt and pepper to taste. Sauté, stirring constantly, for 5 minutes.

5. Add the potatoes, wine, broth, tomato paste, and rosemary. Turn the heat to high, and bring to a boil. Cover the pan, transfer it to the oven, and bake until the meat and potatoes are tender, about 1 hour.

6. Meanwhile, bring a small pot of water to a boil. Add the carrots and cook until tender, 5–7 minutes. Remove with a slotted spoon and reserve. Repeat with the pearl onions.

7. Place the olive oil in a small skillet over medium heat. Add the mushrooms and sauté until tender, about 10 minutes.

8. When the meat is cooked through, transfer the casserole to a burner over medium heat. Add the cooked carrots, pearl onions, and mushrooms, and stir in the currant jelly. Adjust the salt and pepper to taste. Heat through, about 7 minutes, and serve garnished with the parsley.

Yields 15 cups.

GINGER-CRUSTED SALMON

PS LEVEL	SERVING	CALORIES	% FROM FAT	FAT	PROTEIN	CARB.	CHOL.	SODIUM
PS 1	5 oz. salmon with 2 T. each breading and sauce	228	21.3%	5.4 g	29.9 g	9.2 g	74 mg	874 mg
PS 2	6 oz. salmon with 2 T. each breading and sauce	260	22.1%	6.4 g	35.5 g	9.2 g	88 mg	893 mg
PS 3	8 oz. salmon with 3 T. each breading and sauce	358	21.6%	8.6 g	47.6 g	13.8 g	118 mg	1,321 mg

This is an easy and elegant dinner-party dish; stir together the sauce in advance and finish off your side dishes while the salmon bakes.

¹⁄₄ cup low-sodium soy sauce

¹⁄₄ cup plus 4 teaspoons mirin (sweet rice wine), divided

¹⁄₄ cup water

2 teaspoons sugar

¹⁄₄ cup fresh bread crumbs

2 tablespoons prepared horseradish

4 teaspoons minced fresh ginger

³⁄₄ teaspoon salt

¹⁄₂ teaspoon white pepper

4 salmon fillets (each weighing 5 ounces for PS 1, 6 ounces for PS 2, or 8 ounces for PS 3)

1. Preheat the oven to 350 degrees and coat a baking sheet with cooking spray.

2. Whisk together the soy sauce, ¼ cup of the mirin, the water, and the sugar until the sugar is dissolved. Set aside.

3. Place the bread crumbs, horseradish, ginger, 4 teaspoons mirin, salt, and pepper in the bowl of a food processor and process until moistened and well combined.

4. Press 1 tablespoon (PS 1 and 2) or 1½ tablespoons (PS 3) onto each side of each salmon fillet and place on the prepared baking sheet. Bake without turning until the crust is golden brown, about 10 minutes.

5. Serve the salmon drizzled with the reserved sauce.

Yields salmon for 4, ½ cup breading mixture, and ¾ cup sauce.

NOTE: Double the breading mixture if preparing four PS 3 servings.

GREEK FETA CHICKEN

PS LEVEL	SERVING	CALORIES	% FROM FAT	FAT	PROTEIN	CARB.	CHOL.	SODIUM
PS 1	4 oz. chicken with 2 T. topping	138	22.5%	3.4 g	22.7 g	3.1 g	59 mg	342 mg
PS 2	5 oz. chicken with 2 T. topping	163	20.4%	3.7 g	27.9 g	3.1 g	72 mg	357 mg
PS 3	6 oz. chicken with 3 T. topping	207	22.4%	5.2 g	34.0 g	4.7 g	88 mg	513 mg

A tangy topping dresses up chicken breasts for a Mediterranean meal.

4 boneless, skinless chicken breast halves (each weighing 4 ounces for PS 1, 5 ounces for PS 2, or 6 ounces for PS 3)

1 cup fat-free Italian salad dressing

2 ounces feta cheese, crumbled

$\frac{1}{4}$ cup chopped, drained canned artichoke hearts

5 sun-dried tomato halves (not packed in oil), blanched in boiling water until softened and chopped to measure $\frac{1}{4}$ cup

2 tablespoons chopped, pitted black olives (Niçoise or Kalamata)

1$\frac{1}{2}$ teaspoons chopped fresh oregano

1$\frac{1}{2}$ teaspoons chopped fresh parsley

1 tablespoon toasted pine nuts

1. Arrange the chicken breasts in a nonreactive dish and pour the Italian dressing over them. Cover, refrigerate, and marinate at least an hour or up to overnight.

2. Preheat the oven to 350 degrees. Coat a baking pan with cooking spray and arrange the drained chicken in the pan. Bake for 20 minutes.

3. Meanwhile, mix together all the remaining ingredients in a medium bowl.

4. Top each chicken breast with 2 tablespoons (PS 1 and 2) or 3 tablespoons (PS 3) of the feta cheese mixture and return to the oven for 10 minutes more, or until cheese is softened. Serve at once.

Yields chicken for 4 and 1 cup topping.

PIZZA CRUST

This dough makes thin, crispy, California-style pizza—perfect for portion savvy dining! Freeze extra balls of dough, then just thaw and roll for homemade pizza anytime.

¼ cup warm water
1 tablespoon sugar
1 package (¼ ounce) dry yeast
2 tablespoons plain, nonfat yogurt
½ teaspoon salt
¾ cup cool water
3 cups all-purpose flour

1. Combine the ¼ cup warm water with the sugar and yeast in the bowl of an electric mixer or food processor fitted with a dough hook and mix to combine. Let stand until foamy, about 10 minutes.

2. Add the yogurt, salt, and ¾ cup cool water. Mix with the dough hook at medium speed and gradually add flour. Continue mixing and adding flour until the dough pulls from the side of the bowl and has a velvety texture.

3. Turn the dough into a clean bowl and lightly coat the surface with cooking spray. Cover and let rise in a warm place until doubled in volume, about 2 hours. Divide the dough into 8 equal balls weighing 3½ ounces each.

4. Preheat the oven to 400 degrees. For each pizza you wish to make, coat a 12-inch pizza pan with cooking spray. Stretch or roll one ball of dough into a round, then stretch over the prepared pan. Lightly spray with cooking spray, prick the surface several times with a fork, and prebake for 5 minutes.

5. Remove crust from oven to add toppings of choice (see the accompanying recipes or the guidelines in the Portion Savvy Plan). Return to the oven and bake for 10 minutes more until the pizza is bubbling and the crust is golden brown.

Yields 28 ounces of dough to make eight 12-inch pizzas.

PIZZA WITH CHICKEN AND BROCCOLI

PS LEVEL	SERVING	CALORIES	% FROM FAT	FAT	PROTEIN	CARB.	CHOL.	SODIUM
PS 1	2 slices	265	27.8%	8.2 g	26.2 g	22.6 g	52 mg	354 mg
PS 2	3 slices	398	27.8%	12.3 g	39.5 g	33.9 g	78 mg	531 mg
PS 3	4 slices	530	27.8%	16.4 g	52.4 g	45.2 g	104 mg	708 mg

Better than pepperoni—chicken dresses up your pizza without grease.

¼ cup fat-free, reduced-sodium chicken broth

½ onion, sliced thin

1 prebaked 12-inch Pizza Crust (see previous recipe)

2½ ounces shredded part-skim mozzarella cheese, divided

6 ounces cooked skinless chicken breast, thinly sliced

¼ cup low-fat marinara sauce or House Marinara (see recipe on page 197)

1 teaspoon dried oregano

1. Heat the chicken broth in a medium skillet over medium heat, add the onion, and sauté until softened.

2. Sprinkle half the cheese over the pizza crust. Top with the onions, then the chicken, then the marinara sauce. Sprinkle with the remaining cheese and the oregano.

3. Bake the pizza until bubbling and golden brown, 8–10 minutes. *Yields* 6 slices.

TO PORTION: Cut the pizza into 6 slices and serve according to your PS level.

PIZZA WITH FENNEL AND PINE NUTS

PS LEVEL	SERVING	CALORIES	% FROM FAT	FAT	PROTEIN	CARB.	CHOL.	SODIUM
PS 1	2 slices	248	30.5%	8.4 g	20.8 g	23.2 g	28 mg	526 mg
PS 2	3 slices	372	30.5%	12.6 g	31.2 g	34.8 g	42 mg	789 mg
PS 3	4 slices	496	30.5%	16.8 g	41.6 g	46.4 g	56 mg	1,052 mg

Fennel is the unexpected flavor in this delicious combination of caramelized vegetables. Also known as sweet anise, fennel is a white bulb available in the produce department of your supermarket.

¼ cup fat-free, reduced-sodium chicken broth

¼ red onion, julienned

¼ bulb fennel, julienned

1 prebaked 12-inch Pizza Crust (see recipe on page 179)

4 ounces nonfat mozzarella cheese, shredded, divided

½ pound Roma tomatoes, blanched, peeled, seeded, and chopped

2 ounces fontina cheese, shredded

1½ teaspoons fennel seed

1½ tablespoons toasted pine nuts

1. Heat the chicken broth in a medium skillet over medium heat, add the onion and fennel, and sauté until softened.

2. Sprinkle half the mozzarella cheese over the pizza crust. Top with the onions and fennel. Distribute the tomatoes evenly over the pie, then sprinkle with the remaining cheeses, the fennel seed, and the pine nuts.

3. Bake the pizza until bubbling and golden brown, 10–12 minutes.

Yields 6 slices.

TO PORTION: Cut the pizza into 6 slices and serve according to your PS level.

PIZZA WITH SHRIMP, MUSHROOMS, AND RED PEPPER

PS LEVEL	SERVING	CALORIES	% FROM FAT	FAT	PROTEIN	CARB.	CHOL.	SODIUM
PS 1	2 slices	280	31.9%	9.8 g	25.2 g	21.6 g	138 mg	278 mg
PS 2	3 slices	420	31.9%	14.7 g	37.8 g	32.4 g	207 mg	417 mg
PS 3	4 slices	560	31.9%	19.6 g	50.4 g	43.2 g	276 mg	556 mg

Classic California style. Try shiitake mushrooms for an exotic variation.

¼ cup fat-free, reduced-sodium chicken broth

4 ounces mushrooms, sliced

¼ cup dry white wine

8 ounces raw shrimp, peeled and deveined

1 tablespoon minced garlic

1 prebaked 12-inch Pizza Crust (see recipe on page 179)

1 canned roasted red bell pepper, drained, seeded, and cut into ½-inch strips

4 ounces soft goat cheese

¼ teaspoon crushed red pepper

1 teaspoon dried thyme

2 teaspoons chopped fresh basil

1. Heat the chicken broth in a medium skillet over medium heat, add the mushrooms, and sauté until softened. Remove from pan and set aside.

2. Return the skillet to medium-high heat, add the white wine, then add the shrimp and garlic and sauté until the shrimp is just cooked through.

3. Sprinkle the mushrooms over the pizza crust, then cover with red pepper strips placed on the diagonal. Distribute the shrimp evenly around the pizza.

4. Crumble the goat cheese over the top, then sprinkle with the crushed red pepper and the thyme.

5. Bake the pizza until bubbling and golden brown, 8–10 minutes. Sprinkle with the basil and serve.

Yields 6 slices.

TO PORTION: Cut the pizza into 6 slices and serve according to your PS level.

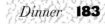

POLENTA LASAGNA

PS LEVEL	SERVING	CALORIES	% FROM FAT	FAT	PROTEIN	CARB.	CHOL.	SODIUM
PS 1	1 piece	284	35.6%	11.0 g	17.1 g	27.8 g	33 mg	740 mg
PS 2 & 3	1½ pieces	426	35.6%	16.5 g	25.7 g	41.7 g	50 mg	1,110 mg

This new take on the well-loved standby substitutes corn polenta for lasagna noodles and creamy goat cheese for ricotta.

12 ounces soft goat cheese

1 teaspoon crushed red pepper

2 pounds frozen spinach, thawed and squeezed dry

2 egg whites

2 pounds prepared polenta, cut into 24 crosswise slices

3 cups low-fat marinara sauce (bottled, or see the House Marinara recipe on page 197)

1½ ounces Parmesan cheese, grated

4 ounces nonfat mozzarella cheese, shredded

½ cup chopped fresh basil

1. Preheat oven to 400 degrees. Coat a 13-by-9-inch baking dish with cooking spray.

2. In a mixing bowl, combine the goat cheese, red pepper flakes, spinach, and egg whites.

3. Arrange 12 of the polenta slices in the baking dish. Top with half the goat cheese mixture, then cover with 1½ cups of the marinara sauce. Repeat with the remaining polenta, cheese mixture, and sauce.

4. Cover the pan with aluminum foil and bake for 40 minutes. Uncover, sprinkle with the Parmesan and mozzarella cheeses, and bake until the cheese is melted and bubbling, about 10 minutes more. Remove from the oven, sprinkle with the basil, let stand for 10 minutes, and serve.

TO PORTION: Cut into 8 pieces, 4 long by 2 wide.

PORK MARBELLA

PS LEVEL	SERVING	CALORIES	% FROM FAT	FAT	PROTEIN	CARB.	CHOL.	SODIUM
PS 1	4 oz. pork with 2 T. sauce	212	23.8%	5.6 g	30.2 g	8.5 g	91 mg	142 mg
PS 2	5 oz. pork with 2 T. sauce	246	24.1%	6.6 g	36.1 g	8.5 g	109 mg	156 mg
PS 3	6 oz. pork with 3 T. sauce	302	23.5%	7.9 g	42.4 g	12.8 g	127 mg	206 mg

Pork naturally marries with the sweet, sour, and salty flavors of a Marbella sauce. Just three steps create a complex dish that will taste as if you've been cooking for hours.

1½ pounds pork tenderloin

¼ cup dry white wine

¼ cup fat-free, reduced-sodium chicken broth

¼ cup chopped, pitted prunes

2 tablespoons plus 2 teaspoons packed brown sugar

2 tablespoons plus 2 teaspoons red wine vinegar

¼ cup chopped, pitted green olives

2 cloves garlic, minced

2 teaspoons dried oregano

2 tablespoons chopped capers

Black pepper to taste

1. Preheat the oven to 400 degrees. Coat a large skillet with cooking spray and sear the pork on all four sides, about 3 minutes per side.

2. Transfer the pork to a roasting dish and roast for 25–30 minutes, until no longer pink and the internal temperature reaches 155 degrees. Cover and let stand for 10 minutes before slicing.

3. Meanwhile, combine the wine, broth, prunes, brown sugar, vinegar, olives, garlic, oregano, capers, and black pepper in a saucepan. Bring to a simmer over medium heat. Simmer gently, uncovered, for 5–10 minutes or until syrupy.

4. Slice the tenderloin into medallions and serve topped with the sauce.

Yields 20 ounces pork tenderloin and 1 cup sauce.

TURKEY STEW

PS LEVEL	SERVING	CALORIES	% FROM FAT	FAT	PROTEIN	CARB.	CHOL.	SODIUM
PS 1	2½ c.	349	21.1%	8.6 g	25.9 g	45.8 g	55 mg	481 mg
PS 2	3 c.	419	21.1%	10.3 g	31.0 g	55.0 g	66 mg	577 mg
PS 3	3½ c.	489	21.1%	12.0 g	36.3 g	64.1 g	77 mg	673 mg

This hearty stew features superfoods of the Americas: turkey, tomatoes, and sweet potatoes.

1½ teaspoons olive oil

1 pound skinless turkey breast, trimmed of fat and cut into 1-inch cubes

1½ cups thinly sliced leeks

1 cup julienned carrot

1 cup fat-free, reduced-sodium chicken broth

1 14½-ounce can diced tomatoes, undrained

1½ teaspoons poultry seasoning

½ teaspoon salt

½ teaspoon coarsely ground black pepper

1 bay leaf

1½ pounds sweet potatoes, peeled and diced

1½ cups frozen corn kernels

1½ cups frozen chopped spinach

1. Heat the oil in a Dutch oven over medium-high heat. Add the turkey and leeks and sauté until browned, about 10 minutes.

2. Add the carrots, broth, tomatoes, poultry seasoning, salt, pepper, and bay leaf. Bring to a boil, reduce heat, cover, and simmer for 1 hour or until the turkey is tender.

3. Add the sweet potatoes, corn, and spinach and simmer, covered, until the sweet potatoes are tender, about 20 minutes. Discard the bay leaf and serve.

Yields 12 cups.

VARIATION: For a vegetarian stew, substitute an additional two pounds of vegetables for the turkey or see "Vegetarian Alternatives" on page 209.

TURKEY TETRAZZINI

PS LEVEL	SERVING	CALORIES	% FROM FAT	FAT	PROTEIN	CARB.	CHOL.	SODIUM
PS 1	1 piece (10 oz.)	345	22.8%	9.2 g	34.2 g	35.8 g	51 mg	499 mg
PS 2	1⅓ pieces (13 oz.)	459	22.8%	12.2 g	45.5 g	47.6 g	68 mg	664 mg
PS 3	1½ pieces (15 oz.)	518	22.8%	13.8 g	51.3 g	53.7 g	77 mg	749 mg

Traditionally a fat and calorie land mine, this tetrazzini has had a modern makeover. It's great for using up Thanksgiving leftovers.

½ pound fettuccine

4 leeks, well washed, dried, and finely chopped

½ pound crimini mushrooms, sliced

1 teaspoon chopped fresh rosemary, divided

¼ cup all-purpose flour

⅔ cup 1% milk

4 cups fat-free, reduced-sodium chicken broth

3 cups cubed cooked turkey breast

1 teaspoon fresh lemon juice

Salt and pepper to taste

4 ounces grated Parmesan cheese

⅓ cup seasoned bread crumbs

4 teaspoons grated lemon zest

4 teaspoons chopped fresh parsley

1. Preheat the oven to 450 degrees. Coat a 13-by-9-inch baking dish with cooking spray.

2. Bring a large pot of water to a boil and cook the fettuccine according to package directions, just until al dente. Drain and set aside.

3. Coat the bottom of a medium saucepan with cooking spray and place over medium heat. Add the leeks and sauté until lightly browned, about 5 minutes. Add the mushrooms and ½ teaspoon of the rosemary and sauté until the mushrooms are softened, about 5 minutes more. Add the flour and cook, stirring, for 1 minute. Gradually stir in the milk, then the broth, and continue to stir until slightly thickened, about 4 minutes.

4. Remove the sauce from the heat and stir in the turkey. Season with the lemon juice, salt, and pepper.

5. Gently combine the turkey mixture with the fettuccine and turn into the prepared baking dish.

6. In a small bowl, combine the Parmesan cheese, bread crumbs, lemon zest, parsley, the remaining ½ teaspoon rosemary, and salt and pepper to taste. Sprinkle over the casserole.

7. Bake the tetrazzini until bubbling and browned, 20–30 minutes.

TO PORTION: Cut the casserole into 8 pieces (4 long by 2 wide) and serve as directed for your PS level; double-check your serving with the scale.

VARIATION: For a vegetarian dish, substitute textured soy protein for the turkey according to the instructions in "Vegetarian Alternatives" on page 209.

SIDES AND SALADS

BUTTERNUT SQUASH PURÉE

PS LEVEL	SERVING	CALORIES	% FROM FAT	FAT	PROTEIN	CARB.	CHOL.	SODIUM
PS 1	½ cup	86	1.8%	0.2 g	1.9 g	22.4 g	0 mg	43 mg
PS 2 & 3	¾ cup	129	1.8%	0.3 g	2.9 g	33.6 g	0 mg	65 mg

Skip the buttery purées served at some popular chains and try this naturally rich version instead.

4 pounds raw butternut squash

2 cups water

Dash cinnamon

Dash nutmeg

Dash garlic powder

Dash salt

Dash white pepper

1. Preheat the oven to 350 degrees. Halve the squash lengthwise, scoop out the seeds, and place the squash cut side down in a roasting pan. Add the water and bake until tender, about 1 hour.

2. Scoop the squash out of the shell and place in a large mixing bowl. Add the seasonings and whip with a hand mixer until smooth.

3. Serve as the carbohydrate side dish for any poultry, meat, or seafood meal.

Yields 4 cups.

CREAMED SPINACH

PS LEVEL	SERVING	CALORIES	% FROM FAT	FAT	PROTEIN	CARB.	CHOL.	SODIUM
PS 1	⅓ cup	43	22.7%	1.3 g	2.8 g	6.7 g	1 mg	101 mg
PS 2 & 3	½ cup	65	22.7%	1.9 g	4.2 g	10.1 g	2 mg	152 mg

Comfort food for your inner child and your outer Popeye.

Béchamel Sauce

1½ cups 1% milk

½ medium onion, cut into ½-inch slices

5 black peppercorns
1 bay leaf
4 teaspoons low-fat margarine
3 tablespoons all-purpose flour
Dash salt
Dash white pepper
Dash nutmeg

1½ pounds fresh spinach, well washed, dried, and stemmed

1. To make the Béchamel Sauce, combine the milk, onion, peppercorns, and bay leaf in a small saucepan. Scald over medium-high heat until small bubbles form around the edge; do not boil. Remove from the heat, cover, and let stand for 10 minutes. Strain through a sieve, reserving the onion solids and discarding the bay leaf and peppercorns. Set aside.

2. Melt the margarine in a heavy saucepan over medium heat. Whisk in the flour and cook 1 minute, stirring constantly. Lower the heat and gradually whisk in the strained milk mixture. Continue to cook, stirring, until the sauce is thickened, about 5 minutes more. Season with salt, white pepper, and nutmeg and keep warm over low heat.

3. Coat a skillet with cooking spray, place over medium heat, and add the reserved onions. Sauté for 1–2 minutes. Add the spinach all at once and continue to sauté until wilted. Stir the spinach into the Béchamel Sauce and season with additional salt and white pepper to taste.

4. Serve as a vegetable side dish to any poultry, meat, or seafood meal.

Yields 4 cups.

CUCUMBER SALAD

PS LEVEL	SERVING	CALORIES	% FROM FAT	FAT	PROTEIN	CARB.	CHOL.	SODIUM
PS 1–3	½ cup	43	31.6%	1.6 g	0.6 g	7.3 g	0 mg	3 mg

Try this Asian refresher on a hot summer day.

1 pound English (hothouse) cucumbers
½ cup finely shredded green cabbage
2 teaspoons sesame oil
1 tablespoon minced fresh ginger
1 teaspoon minced garlic
2 tablespoons sugar
¼ cup seasoned rice vinegar

1. Trim the ends off the cucumbers. Using a vegetable peeler or zester, remove lengthwise strips of skin so that the cucumbers look striped. Slice into rounds ¼ inch thick and place in a nonreactive mixing bowl. Add the cabbage.

2. Heat the sesame oil in a small skillet until hot. Remove from the heat, add the ginger and garlic, and quickly stir so that the garlic does not brown. Dissolve the sugar in the rice vinegar and add to the ginger mixture, stirring to combine.

3. Pour the dressing over the cucumber and cabbage and toss lightly. Cover and refrigerate for at least one hour and up to overnight. The flavor will improve with time.

Yields 3 cups.

JICAMA SLAW

PS LEVEL	SERVING	CALORIES	% FROM FAT	FAT	PROTEIN	CARB.	CHOL.	SODIUM
PS 1–3	½ cup	47	2.6%	0.2 g	0.8 g	11.7 g	0 mg	28 mg

Jicama stands in for cabbage in a slightly sweet slaw that cozies up to a burger with ease.

1½ cups peeled, grated jicama
¾ cup peeled, grated carrots
¾ cup peeled, grated Granny Smith apples
¼ cup frozen apple juice concentrate, thawed
¼ cup cider vinegar

2 teaspoons Dijon mustard

2 cloves garlic, minced

¼ cup currants

1. Combine the jicama, carrots, and apples in a mixing bowl. In a small bowl, stir together the apple juice concentrate, vinegar, mustard, garlic, and currants. Pour the dressing over the jicama mixture and toss well. Chill until ready to serve.

Yields 3 cups.

MUSTARD POTATOES

PS LEVEL	SERVING	CALORIES	% FROM FAT	FAT	PROTEIN	CARB.	CHOL.	SODIUM
PS 1	6 wedges (½ cup)	118	5.7%	0.8 g	3.5 g	25.5 g	0 mg	159 mg
PS 2 & 3	9 wedges (¾ cup)	177	5.7%	1.2 g	5.3 g	38.3 g	0 mg	239 mg

With mustard and spices jazzing up the flavor, who needs oil?

½ cup Dijon mustard

2 teaspoons paprika

1 teaspoon ground cumin

1 teaspoon garlic powder

16 small to medium new red potatoes (about 3 pounds), skins pricked with a fork and cut into quarters

1. Preheat the oven to 400 degrees and coat a roasting pan with cooking spray.

2. Blend the mustard, paprika, cumin, and garlic powder in a mixing bowl. Add the potatoes and toss to coat evenly.

3. Turn the potatoes into the roasting pan and bake until tender, about 1 hour.

4. Serve as the carbohydrate side dish to any poultry, meat, or seafood meal.

Yields 5 cups.

ORANGE COUSCOUS

PS LEVEL	SERVING	CALORIES	% FROM FAT	FAT	PROTEIN	CARB.	CHOL.	SODIUM
PS 1	½ cup	108	1.4%	0.2 g	6.2 g	21.9 g	0 mg	23 mg
PS 2 & 3	¾ cup	162	1.4%	0.3 g	9.3 g	32.9 g	0 mg	34 mg

Couscous is flaked wheat that's already been cooked, so it's quick as can be!

2 cups fat-free, reduced-sodium chicken broth or water
1½ cups raw couscous
1½ teaspoons grated orange zest
Dash allspice

1. Bring the broth or water to a boil in a medium saucepan. Remove from the heat and stir in the couscous, orange zest, and all-spice. Cover and let stand for 5 minutes.

2. Uncover and fluff with a fork. Serve as the carbohydrate side dish to any poultry, meat, or seafood meal.

Yields 5 cups.

PAPAYA RICE

PS LEVEL	SERVING	CALORIES	% FROM FAT	FAT	PROTEIN	CARB.	CHOL.	SODIUM
PS 1	½ cup	121	2.0%	0.3 g	3.9 g	27.2 g	0 mg	217 mg
PS 2 & 3	¾ cup	182	2.0%	0.5 g	5.9 g	40.8 g	0 mg	326 mg

This intriguing pilaf will transport your palate to the tropics.

½ onion, diced
2 teaspoons minced fresh ginger
1 clove garlic, minced
¼ teaspoon ground cardamom
½ cup papaya nectar
½ cup fat-free, reduced-sodium chicken broth
½ cup basmati or jasmine rice, rinsed and drained
¼ teaspoon salt
¾ cup peeled, diced papaya

1. Coat the bottom of a saucepan with cooking spray and place over medium heat. Add the onion, ginger, and garlic and sauté for 1 minute. Add the cardamom and stir.

2. Add the papaya nectar, chicken broth, rice, and salt. Bring to a boil, add papaya, and reduce heat to low. Cover and cook for 10 minutes.

3. Remove from the heat and let stand, covered, for 15 minutes. Uncover and fluff with a fork.

4. Serve as the carbohydrate side dish to any poultry, meat, or seafood meal.

Yields 2 cups.

ROASTED ROOT VEGETABLES

PS LEVEL	SERVING	CALORIES	% FROM FAT	FAT	PROTEIN	CARB.	CHOL.	SODIUM
PS 1	½ cup	49	2.9%	0.2 g	1.6 g	11.8 g	0 mg	43 mg
PS 2 & 3	¾ cup	74	2.9%	0.3 g	2.4 g	17.7 g	0 mg	65 mg

Try this hearty side dish to warm up a winter supper.

1 pound carrots, peeled and quartered
½ pound turnips, peeled and quartered
½ pound rutabagas, peeled and quartered
⅓ cup fat-free, reduced-sodium chicken broth
4 teaspoons thawed frozen apple juice concentrate
4 teaspoons honey
1 teaspoon balsamic vinegar
1 teaspoon grated lemon rind

1. Preheat the oven to 350 degrees. Coat a 13-by-9-inch baking dish with cooking spray and scatter the vegetables inside. Mist them with a little more spray.

2. In a small bowl, combine the broth, apple juice, honey, vinegar, and lemon zest. Drizzle over the vegetables.

3. Cover the pan with foil and bake until tender, about 40 to 50 minutes. Uncover and bake 10 minutes more to brown.

4. Serve as the vegetable side dish to any poultry, meat, or seafood meal.

Yields 4 cups.

WILD RICE PILAF

PS LEVEL	SERVING	CALORIES	% FROM FAT	FAT	PROTEIN	CARB.	CHOL.	SODIUM
PS 1	½ cup	112	13.1%	2.0 g	9.8 g	19.8 g	0 mg	259 mg
PS 2 & 3	¾ cup	168	13.1%	3.0 g	14.7 g	29.7 g	0 mg	389 mg

With an earthy flavor and a generous helping of fiber, this makes a great side to any meat or seafood dish.

1 tablespoon olive oil
1 cup chopped mushrooms
1 cup chopped onions
½ cup wild rice
½ cup barley
2 cloves garlic, minced
1 teaspoon chopped fresh thyme
4 cups fat-free, reduced-sodium chicken broth
½ teaspoon salt

1. Heat the oil in a large saucepan over medium heat. Add the mushrooms and onions and sauté until browned, about 5 minutes.

2. Add the wild rice, barley, garlic, and thyme and sauté for 1 minute more.

3. Add the chicken broth and salt and bring to a boil. Reduce to a simmer, cover, and cook until the liquid is absorbed, about 45 minutes. Let stand, covered, until ready to serve.

4. Serve as a carbohydrate side dish to any poultry, meat, or seafood meal.

Yields 4 cups.

SAUCES, RUBS, AND DRESSINGS

ARTICHOKE PESTO

PS LEVEL	SERVING	CALORIES	% FROM FAT	FAT	PROTEIN	CARB.	CHOL.	SODIUM
PS 1 & 2	2 T.	20	30.5%	0.7 g	1.3 g	2.5 g	1 mg	44 mg
PS 3	3 T.	30	30.5%	1.1 g	2.0 g	3.8 g	1.5 mg	66 mg

See Asparagus, Lima Bean, and Bow-Tie Pasta Salad on page 164.

HERB VINAIGRETTE

PS LEVEL	SERVING	CALORIES	% FROM FAT	FAT	PROTEIN	CARB.	CHOL.	SODIUM
PS 1–3	2 T.	14	46.4 %	1.0 g	1.0 g	1.4 g	0 mg	24 mg

Pour on the fresh herbs, add just a splash of olive oil—and you'll never go back to high-fat, sodium-loaded bottled dressings.

1 cup fat-free, reduced-sodium chicken broth

6 tablespoons fresh lemon juice

6 tablespoons red wine vinegar

1½ tablespoons Dijon mustard

1 tablespoon olive oil

2 cloves garlic

2 teaspoons finely chopped fresh parsley

2 teaspoons finely chopped fresh basil

1 teaspoon finely chopped fresh chives

1 teaspoon finely chopped fresh dill

1 teaspoon finely chopped fresh thyme

2 tablespoons finely chopped shallots

Salt and pepper

1. Combine all the ingredients but the shallots in a blender or food processor and process until smooth. Add the shallots and process a few seconds more. Season to taste with salt and pepper.

Yields 2 cups.

HONEY-CHILI SAUCE

PS LEVEL	SERVING	CALORIES	% FROM FAT	FAT	PROTEIN	CARB.	CHOL.	SODIUM
PS 1 & 2	2 T.	104	6.9%	1.0 g	2.8 g	25.2 g	0 mg	20 mg
PS 3	3 T.	156	6.9%	1.5 g	4.2 g	37.8 g	0 mg	30 mg

A sweet hit of spice from south of the border.

¼ cup finely chopped shallots

⅔ cup honey, slightly warmed

¼ cup sherry vinegar

1½ cups fat-free, reduced-sodium chicken broth

1 tablespoon chopped seeded dried pasilla chili

¼ teaspoon cumin

1 teaspoon chopped fresh cilantro

Salt and pepper to taste

3 tablespoons chopped toasted pecans

1. Coat the bottom of a small saucepan with cooking spray and place over medium-high heat. Add the chopped shallots and sauté until browned, 5 to 10 minutes.

2. Carefully add the honey and vinegar to the pan; the mixture will foam up. Quickly stir in the broth, chili, and cumin, bring to a boil, and reduce the sauce by half.

3. Purée the sauce in a food processor or blender until smooth. Return to a clean pan and keep warm until ready to serve.

4. At serving time, add the chopped cilantro and season to taste with salt and pepper. Stir in the pecans and serve over poultry, seafood, or meat.

Yields 1 cup.

HOUSE MARINARA

PS LEVEL	SERVING	CALORIES	% FROM FAT	FAT	PROTEIN	CARB.	CHOL.	SODIUM
PS 1	¾ cup	73	22.0%	1.8 g	2.3 g	11.9 g	0 mg	307 mg
PS 2	1 cup	97	22.0%	2.4 g	3.1 g	15.9 g	0 mg	409 mg
PS 3	1¼ cups	121	22.0%	3.0 g	3.9 g	19.9 g	0 mg	511 mg

Cook up a batch of this aromatic sauce every weekend and many of your weekly mealtime challenges will be solved.

Fat-free, reduced-sodium chicken broth as needed for sautéing

2 cups diced onions

1½ teaspoons minced garlic

½ cup dry red wine

4 pounds chopped canned tomatoes, undrained

2 tablespoons maple sugar

1 tablespoon olive oil

2 tablespoons chopped fresh basil

2 tablespoons chopped fresh oregano

2 tablespoons chopped fresh Italian parsley

Dash salt

1. Heat 2 tablespoons chicken broth in a stock pot over medium heat. Add the onions and sauté, adding broth in 2-tablespoon increments as the liquid evaporates, until the onions are caramelized, about 15 minutes.

2. Add the garlic and sauté 5 minutes more. Add the red wine and cook for 5 to 10 minutes to evaporate the alcohol.

3. Add the tomatoes, maple sugar, and olive oil. Return the sauce to a simmer and continue to cook for 30 minutes. Stir in the herbs and salt. Serve over pasta.

VARIATION: If you prefer a smooth sauce, purée in a food processor before serving.

Yields 8 cups.

LEMON-CUMIN RUB

PS LEVEL	SERVING	CALORIES	% FROM FAT	FAT	PROTEIN	CARB.	CHOL.	SODIUM
PS 1–3	1 T.	13	11.4%	0.2 g	0.4 g	3.1 g	0 mg	121 mg

Rubs infuse flavor directly into the meat and are low in calories too!

1 tablespoon cumin seed

¼ cup dried onion

2 tablespoons dried parsley

1 teaspoon sugar

½ teaspoon white peppercorns

½ teaspoon kosher salt

1 tablespoon grated lemon zest

3 tablespoons fresh lemon juice

1. Toast the cumin seeds in a small, nonstick skillet over low heat until fragrant; be careful not to burn them.

2. In a spice or coffee grinder, combine the cumin with the onion, parsley, sugar, peppercorns, and salt. Grind to a powder.

3. Stir together the spice mixture and the lemon zest and juice.

4. Rub 1 tablespoon of the mixture into each serving of poultry, seafood, or pork, let marinate for one hour in the refrigerator, then grill, roast, or bake until cooked through.

Yields ½ cup.

LIME-SOY VINAIGRETTE

PS LEVEL	SERVING	CALORIES	% FROM FAT	FAT	PROTEIN	CARB.	CHOL.	SODIUM
PS 1–3	2 T.	20	46.8%	1.2 g	0.4 g	2.4 g	0 mg	242 mg

Try this Asian-inspired dressing for a low-fat Chinese chicken salad.

1 cup rice vinegar

½ cup low-sodium soy sauce

½ cup fresh lime juice

4 teaspoons dark sesame oil

2 teaspoons lemon zest

2 teaspoons minced fresh ginger

4 cloves garlic, minced

1. Combine all ingredients in a blender or food processor and process until smooth.

Yields 2 cups.

MARBELLA SAUCE

PS LEVEL	SERVING	CALORIES	% FROM FAT	FAT	PROTEIN	CARB.	CHOL.	SODIUM
PS 1 & 2	2 T.	42	11.8%	0.6 g	0.7 g	8.5 g	0 mg	72 mg
PS 3	3 T.	63	11.8%	0.9 g	1.1 g	12.8 g	0 mg	108 mg

See Pork Marbella on page 184.

MUSTARD CREAM SAUCE

PS LEVEL	SERVING	CALORIES	% FROM FAT	FAT	PROTEIN	CARB.	CHOL.	SODIUM
PS 1 & 2	2 T.	86	7.0%	0.4 g	4.0 g	6.8 g	0 mg	272 mg
PS 3	3 T.	129	7.0%	0.6 g	6.0 g	10.2 g	0 mg	408 mg

This versatile sauce is equally happy on poultry, meat, or seafood.

4 shallots, chopped

1¼ cups fat-free, reduced-sodium chicken broth, divided

1¼ cups sweet vermouth

½ teaspoon arrowroot

½ cup evaporated skim milk

¼ cup three-grain Dijon mustard

½ teaspoon salt

Dash white pepper

1 tablespoon chopped chives for garnish

1. Coat the bottom of a saucepan with cooking spray and place over medium heat. Add the shallots and sauté until tender, using ¼ cup of the broth to deglaze the pan as necessary.

2. Stir in the remaining broth and the vermouth. Simmer until reduced by three-quarters.

3. Dissolve the arrowroot in a little cold water and add to the pan. Stir until slightly thickened.

4. Transfer the sauce to a food processor or blender. Add the evaporated milk, mustard, salt, and pepper and process until smooth.

5. Serve over poultry, meat, or seafood with the chives as garnish.

Yields 1 cup.

PAPAYA MARINADE

See Southwestern Chicken Salad on page 169.

PAPAYA VINAIGRETTE

PS LEVEL	SERVING	CALORIES	% FROM FAT	FAT	PROTEIN	CARB.	CHOL.	SODIUM
PS 1–3	2 T.	8	0%	0 g	0 g	2.4 g	0 mg	0 mg

Papaya thickens this fat-free dressing— and infuses it with antioxidant beta- carotene.

1½ cups peeled, chopped papaya

¼ cup rice vinegar

2 tablespoons frozen pineapple juice concentrate, thawed

2 tablespoons raspberry vinegar

1 tablespoon fresh lime juice

1 teaspoon chopped fresh mint

¼ teaspoon chili powder

Black pepper to taste

1. Combine all ingredients in a blender or food processor and process until smooth.

Yields 2 cups.

VARIATION: Substitute mango or kiwi for the papaya.

PORT WINE SAUCE

PS LEVEL	SERVING	CALORIES	% FROM FAT	FAT	PROTEIN	CARB.	CHOL.	SODIUM
PS 1 & 2	2 T.	79	0.8%	0 g	2.6 g	13.4 g	0 mg	240 mg
PS 3	3 T.	119	0.8%	0 g	3.9 g	20.1 g	0 mg	360 mg

Try this on roasted pork tenderloin or grilled chicken.

¾ cup port wine

¾ cup low-sodium beef broth

¼ cup frozen cranberry juice concentrate, thawed

½ cup dried cherries

½ teaspoon chopped fresh thyme

½ cup minced shallots

3 cloves garlic, minced

1 teaspoon ground allspice

½ teaspoon salt
¼ teaspoon cracked black peppercorns

1. Combine the port, broth, cranberry juice concentrate, dried cherries, and thyme in a small saucepan. Bring to a rolling boil. Remove from the heat and set aside.

2. Coat a medium skillet with cooking spray and place over medium heat. Add the shallots and garlic and sauté until browned, about 5 to 10 minutes. Add the wine mixture, allspice, salt, and peppercorns. Simmer over low heat until sauce is reduced by half, about 30 minutes.

3. Serve over poultry or meat.

Yields 1 cup.

RASPBERRY VINAIGRETTE

PS LEVEL	SERVING	CALORIES	% FROM FAT	FAT	PROTEIN	CARB.	CHOL.	SODIUM
PS 1–3	2 T.	30	7.4%	0.2 g	0.4 g	7.4 g	0 mg	38 mg

Make your salad special in the summer months, when raspberries are in season.

¾ cup frozen raspberries (not in syrup), thawed
6 tablespoons seasoned rice vinegar
3 tablespoons honey mustard
3 tablespoons honey
3 tablespoons water
3 tablespoons chopped fresh mint leaves
1 shallot
½ cup fresh raspberries

1. Combine all the ingredients except the fresh raspberries in a blender or food processor and process until smooth. Add the fresh raspberries and process briefly to a chunky texture.

Yields 2 cups.

VARIATION: The vinaigrette can also be used as a marinade for poultry, pork, or seafood.

ROSEMARY RUB

PS LEVEL	SERVING	CALORIES	% FROM FAT	FAT	PROTEIN	CARB.	CHOL.	SODIUM
PS 1–3	1 T.	4	23.5%	0.1 g	0.2 g	0.7 g	0 mg	470 mg

The piney flavor of rosemary suggests the south of France.

¼ cup chopped fresh rosemary
1 tablespoon cracked black peppercorns
½ teaspoon cracked white peppercorns
2 teaspoons kosher salt
1 teaspoon dry mustard
1 teaspoon dried oregano
1 teaspoon garlic powder

1. Combine all the ingredients in a small bowl.
2. Rub 1 tablespoon of the mixture into each serving of meat, poultry, or seafood. Marinate for 1 hour in the refrigerator, then grill, roast, or bake until cooked through.
   Yields ½ cup.

SALSA FRESCA

Unlimited condiment; use as desired.

See the Vegetarian Burrito recipe on page 173.

YOGURT SAUCE

PS LEVEL	SERVING	CALORIES	% FROM FAT	FAT	PROTEIN	CARB.	CHOL.	SODIUM
PS 1	¼ c.	41	3.9%	0.2 g	3.2 g	6.9 g	2 mg	115 mg
PS 2	⅓ c.	55	3.9%	0.3 g	4.3 g	9.2 g	3 mg	153 mg
PS 3	6 T.	62	3.9%	0.3 g	4.8 g	10.4 g	3 mg	173 mg

See the Tabbouleh and Tomato Pilaf recipe on page 172.

DESSERTS

Each dessert counts as a snack on the Portion Savvy Plan.

APPLE COBBLER

PS LEVEL	SERVING	CALORIES	% FROM FAT	FAT	PROTEIN	CARB.	CHOL.	SODIUM
PS 1–3	1 piece	106	6.9%	0.8 g	1.0 g	24.6 g	0 mg	64 mg

This dessert makes a great excuse to get another serving of fruit into your day!

3 tablespoons fresh lemon juice

¹/₃ cup instant tapioca

5 Granny Smith apples, peeled, cored, and sliced

¹/₄ cup plus 2¹/₂ teaspoons firmly packed brown sugar, divided

¹/₄ cup plus 1 teaspoon all-purpose flour, divided

¹/₄ teaspoon cinnamon

Dash nutmeg

¹/₂ cup quick-cooking oatmeal

¹/₄ cup granulated sugar

1 tablespoon reduced-fat margarine, softened

3 tablespoons frozen apple juice concentrate, thawed

1. Preheat the oven to 325 degrees. Coat a 13-by-9-inch baking dish with cooking spray.

2. Combine the lemon juice and tapioca in a mixing bowl and mix in the sliced apples. Add 2¹/₂ teaspoons of the brown sugar, 1 teaspoon of the flour, and the cinnamon and nutmeg. Combine well and turn into the pan.

3. In a small bowl, combine the oatmeal, remaining sugars, remaining flour, and margarine and crumble together with your fingers. Add the apple juice concentrate and combine with your fingers to form a coarse meal. Pat over the fruit and bake until bubbly and browned, about 40 minutes. Cool and cut into 12 pieces.

Yields 12 servings.

VARIATION: Substitute 5 cups of assorted berries for the apples.

TO PORTION: Make 3 crosswise and 2 lengthwise cuts.

CARAMEL BARS

PS LEVEL	SERVING	CALORIES	% FROM FAT	FAT	PROTEIN	CARB.	CHOL.	SODIUM
PS 1–3	1 bar	122	19.7%	2.7 g	1.6 g	23.1 g	0 mg	97 mg

Rich and gooey, a portion savvy treat.

1¾ cups plus ¼ cup all-purpose flour, divided
1¾ cups quick-cooking oats
¾ cup firmly packed brown sugar
½ teaspoon baking soda
¼ teaspoon salt
½ cup Date Purée (see recipe on page 206)
2 tablespoons canola oil
2 tablespoons water
¾ cup mini semisweet chocolate chips
½ cup fat-free caramel topping

1. Preheat the oven to 350 degrees. Coat a 13-by-9-inch baking pan with cooking spray.

2. Combine the 1¾ cups flour, the oatmeal, brown sugar, baking soda, and salt in a mixing bowl. Add the Date Purée, oil, and water and combine with your hands until evenly moistened and crumbly.

3. Set aside 1 cup of the oatmeal mixture for the topping. Press the remainder evenly into the bottom of the prepared baking pan. Bake for 10 minutes. Remove from the oven and let cool for 10 minutes.

4. Sprinkle the cooled crust with the chocolate chips. Stir the remaining ¼ cup flour into the caramel topping and drizzle over the chips to within ¼ inch of the edges of the pan. Sprinkle with the reserved oatmeal mixture.

5. Bake for 10 minutes, or until edges are golden brown. Cool and cut into bars.

Yields 32 bars.

TO PORTION: Make 3 lengthwise and 7 crosswise cuts, all evenly spaced.

CHOCOLATE-ORANGE BISCOTTI

PS LEVEL	SERVING	CALORIES	% FROM FAT	FAT	PROTEIN	CARB.	CHOL.	SODIUM
PS 1–3	2 biscotti	138	15.9%	2.4 g	2.6 g	27.0 g	14 mg	92 mg

These crunchy cookies make a sophisticated close to any meal. To do as the Italians do, dunk them in coffee.

1½ cups all-purpose flour
1¼ teaspoons baking powder
¼ teaspoon salt
1½ tablespoons low-fat margarine, softened
¾ cup sugar
1 teaspoon vanilla extract
1 egg
2 egg whites, divided
¼ cup mini semisweet chocolate chips
¼ cup chopped orange zest

1. Preheat the oven to 350 degrees. Line a baking sheet with parchment or waxed paper.
2. Sift the flour, baking powder, and salt together into a small bowl.
3. In a mixing bowl, cream the margarine, sugar, and vanilla together until light and fluffy. Beat in the egg and 1 egg white. By hand, mix in the flour mixture, then the chocolate chips and orange zest.
4. Shape the dough into a log, place on the prepared baking sheet, and press flat. Whisk the remaining egg white with a fork and brush over the dough. Bake for 25 minutes or until lightly browned. Remove from the oven and cool for 10 minutes.
5. Decrease the oven temperature to 200 degrees. Transfer the log to a cutting board and use a serrated knife to cut into 25 slices. Arrange the slices on the baking sheet and bake for 20 minutes, or until golden brown.
Yields 25 cookies.

DATE PURÉE

The sweetness of dates works perfectly for bars, brownies, and cookies; substitute for butter or margarine in any baking recipe.

1 pound pitted dates
1½ cups water
½ teaspoon vanilla extract

1. Combine the dates and the water in a saucepan and cook over low heat for 10 to 15 minutes, until dates are soft. Or cook in the microwave, in a covered, microwave-safe dish, for 5 minutes on high.

2. Transfer to a food processor and purée until smooth. Add the vanilla and purée 1 minute more.

3. Use in portion savvy dessert recipes.

MOLASSES COOKIES

PS LEVEL	SERVING	CALORIES	% FROM FAT	FAT	PROTEIN	CARB.	CHOL.	SODIUM
PS 1–3	2 cookies	96	14.7%	1.6 g	1.4 g	19.6 g	0 mg	120 mg

Try these on a crisp fall day and watch people follow their noses to your kitchen.

1⅓ cups all-purpose flour
1 teaspoon baking soda
½ teaspoon cinnamon
½ teaspoon ginger
Dash cloves
Dash salt
¼ cup low-fat margarine, softened
½ cup firmly packed brown sugar
2 tablespoons molasses
1 egg white
¼ cup granulated sugar

1. In a small bowl, combine the flour, baking soda, cinnamon, ginger, cloves, and salt.

2. Place the margarine, brown sugar, molasses, and egg white in the bowl of a food processor and mix until blended. Add the dry ingredients and process, scraping the sides of the bowl. Gently form the mixture into a ball, wrap in plastic wrap, and chill for 2 hours.

3. Preheat the oven to 375 degrees. Coat two baking sheets with cooking spray.

4. Place the granulated sugar in a small bowl and fill another bowl with water. Roll the dough into thirty-two ¾-inch balls; dip each ball in the water and shake to remove excess moisture, then roll in the sugar. Place 3 inches apart on the baking sheets. Bake for 10 minutes.

5. Remove the cookies to a wire rack and cool.

Yields 32 cookies.

OATMEAL CHOCOLATE CHIP COOKIES

PS LEVEL	SERVING	CALORIES	% FROM FAT	FAT	PROTEIN	CARB.	CHOL.	SODIUM
PS 1–3	2 cookies	92	34.1%	3.6 g	1.6 g	14.2 g	0 mg	66 mg

No life is complete without chocolate chip cookies. Is it?

¼ cup low-fat margarine, softened
¼ cup Date Purée (see recipe on page 206)
3 tablespoons firmly packed brown sugar
1 egg white
1 tablespoon 1% milk
½ cup all-purpose flour
½ cup quick-cooking oatmeal
½ teaspoon cinnamon
¼ teaspoon baking soda
¼ cup mini semisweet chocolate chips

1. Preheat the oven to 350 degrees and coat two baking sheets with cooking spray.

2. In a mixing bowl, cream together the margarine, Date Purée, and brown sugar. Blend in the egg white and milk.

3. In a small bowl, combine the flour, oatmeal, cinnamon, and baking soda.

4. Stir the flour mixture into the margarine mixture. Stir in the chocolate chips.

5. Drop the dough onto the prepared baking sheets by 2½-teaspoonfuls. Press flat.

6. Bake the cookies just until firm on top, 6 to 8 minutes. Let stand for a few minutes, remove to racks, and cool completely.

Yields 24 cookies.

WHITE CHOCOLATE MERINGUE DROPS

PS LEVEL	SERVING	CALORIES	% FROM FAT	FAT	PROTEIN	CARB.	CHOL.	SODIUM
PS 1–3	2 cookies	86	31.7%	3.2 g	1.4 g	13.8 g	0 mg	26 mg

Meringues are easy once you get the hang of whipping the egg whites. These cookies tend to take on different shapes depending upon the weather on the day you bake them—but they always taste great!

3 egg whites

Dash cream of tartar

½ cup sugar

2 teaspoons vanilla extract

½ cup mini white chocolate chips

1. Preheat the oven to 250 degrees. Line two baking sheets with parchment or waxed paper.

2. In a large bowl, beat the egg whites with the cream of tartar at high speed until they hold peaks. Beat in the sugar 1 tablespoon at a time, then beat in the vanilla. Fold in the chips with a rubber spatula.

3. Drop the mixture by level tablespoons onto the prepared baking sheets, 1 inch apart. Bake for 1 hour. Turn off the oven and allow cookies to dry inside for 2 hours more.

Yields 25 cookies.

VEGETARIAN ALTERNATIVES

Each of the alternatives below can substitute for the following ingredients in any portion savvy meal. If your recipe calls for

	PS 1	PS 2	PS 3
Poultry or meat	4 oz.	5 oz.	6 oz.
Seafood	5 oz.	6 oz.	8 oz.

these are the equivalents:

	PS 1	PS 2	PS 3
Tofu	6 oz.	9 oz.	12 oz.
Soy beverage	1 c.	$1\frac{1}{4}$ c.	$1\frac{1}{2}$ c.
Soy-based protein powder	2 T.	3 T.	4 T.
Textured soy protein	4 T.	5 T.	6 T.
Rice and beans	$\frac{1}{4}$ c. each	$\frac{1}{3}$ c. each	$\frac{1}{2}$ c. each
Egg whites	6	9	12
Low-fat cheese	$1\frac{1}{2}$ oz.	2 oz.	$2\frac{1}{2}$ oz.
Nonfat milk	$1\frac{1}{4}$ c.	$1\frac{1}{2}$ c.	2 c.
Nonfat yogurt	1 c.	$1\frac{1}{2}$ c.	$1\frac{3}{4}$ c.

THE PORTION SAVVY SNACK LIST

Each Portion Savvy Snack should have about 100–120 calories and no more than 3 grams of fat per serving. Avoid all foods that contain hydrogenated oils or artificial sweeteners (NutraSweet, etc.).

PS 1 = 2 per day
PS 2 = 3 per day
PS 3 = 4 per day

- 1 small apple, pear, or orange
- ¼ melon (honeydew, cantaloupe, or watermelon)
- ½ grapefruit
- ½ banana
- ¼ papaya or mango
- 15 grapes
- 15 cherries
- 1 cup pineapple
- 1 cup applesauce
- ¾ cup mixed berries
- 6 ounces fruit juice
- 1 ounce dried fruit
- 3 cups lite popcorn (microwaved or air-popped)
- 1 ounce low-fat bagel, potato, or tortilla chips
- 2 medium sourdough pretzels (1 ounce)
- 2 large low-fat rice cakes

- ➤ ½ ounce low-fat crackers with 1½ ounces of low-fat cheese
- ➤ ½ ounce low-fat crackers with 1 teaspoon peanut, almond, or soy butter
- ➤ 1 ounce of ahi or turkey jerky
- ➤ 4 ounces of low-fat pudding
- ➤ 4 ounces of nonfat, fruit-sweetened yogurt
- ➤ 4 vines of red or black licorice
- ➤ 1 low-fat granola or snack bar
- ➤ ½ supplement bar
- ➤ 1 low-fat frozen yogurt bar or frozen fruit bar
- ➤ 4 ounces low-fat frozen yogurt or low-fat ice cream
- ➤ 8 ounces of vanilla-flavored soy or rice milk
- ➤ 1 can (12 ounces) sweetened iced tea, natural soda, lemonade, or limeade
- ➤ 4 ounces red or white wine, or 12 ounces lite beer
- ➤ 1 cappuccino or café latte with nonfat milk
- ➤ Any Portion Savvy Recipe dessert

NOTE: BEVERAGES ARE *NOT* FREE FOODS!

NOTES

1. Lauren J. Nelson and Hamid Hekmat, "Promoting Healthy Nutritional Habits by Paradigmatic Behavior Therapy," *Journal of Behavior Therapy and Experimental Psychiatry* 22/4 (1991): 291–98; J. Polivy and C. P. Herman, "Diagnosis and Treatment of Normal Eating," *Journal of Consulting and Clinical Psychology* 55 (1987): 635–44; G. T. Wilson, "Behavior Modification and the Treatment of Obesity," in A. J. Stunkard, ed., *Obesity* (Philadelphia, Pa.: Saunders, 1980).

2. S. A. Bingham, "The Dietary Assessment of Individuals: Methods, Accuracy, New Techniques and Recommendations," *Nutrition Abstracts and Reviews* 57 (1987): 705–42; A. E. Black et al., "Critical Evaluation of Energy Intake Data Using Fundamental Principles of Energy Physiology: 2. Evaluating the Results of Published Surveys," *European Journal of Clinical Nutrition* 45 (1991): 583–99; A. E. Black et al., "Measurements of Total Energy Expenditure Provide Insights into the Validity of Dietary Measurements of Energy Intake," *Journal of the American Dietetic Association* 93 (1993): 572–79; J. Haraldsdottir, "Minimizing Error in the Field: Quality Control in Dietary Surveys," *European Journal of Clinical Nutrition* 47 (suppl. S2, 1993): S19–24; D. A. Schoeller, "How Accurate Is Self-Reported Dietary Energy Intake?" *Nutrition Reviews* 48 (1990): 373–79.

3. Lori G. Borrud, Cecilia W. Enns, and Sharon L. Mickle, "Changes in Food Consumption Over Time: Continuing Survey of Food Intakes by Individuals 1994 and Nationwide Food Consumption Survey 1977–78," United States Department of Agriculture ARS Report No. 72163, 1996.

4. Ronette R. Briefel et al., "Total Energy Intake of the U.S. Population: The Third National Health and Nutrition Examination Survey, 1988–1991," *American Journal of Clinical Nutrition* 62 (suppl., 1995): 1072S–80S.

5. "Increasing Prevalence of Overweight Among U.S. Adults: The National Health and Nutrition Examination Surveys 1960–1991," *Journal of the American Medical Association* (July 20, 1994): 205–11.

6. D. G. Schlundt et al., "Randomized Evaluation of a Low Fat Ad Libitum Carbohydrate Diet for Weight Reduction," *International Journal of Obesity and Related Metabolic Disorders* 17/11 (1993): 623–29.

7. Frank I. Katch and William D. McArdle, *Introduction to Nutrition, Exercise, and Health,* 4th ed. (Philadelphia/London: Lead Febiger, 1993).

8. J. M. Bryson et al., "Changes in Glucose and Lipid Metabolism Following Weight Loss Produced by a Very Low Calorie Diet in Obese Subjects," *International Journal of Obesity and Related Metabolic Disorders* 20/4 (1996): 338–45; F. Capstick et al., "Very Low Calorie Diet (VLCD): A Useful Alternative in the Treatment of the Obese NIDDM Patient," *Diabetes Research and Clinical Practice* 36/2 (1997): 105–11; M. A. Lane et al., "Diet Restriction in Rhesus Monkeys Lowers Fasting and Glucose-Stimulated Glucoregulatory End Points," *American Journal of Physiology* 268/5 (pt. 1, 1995): E941–48; M. A. Lane et al., "Calorie Restriction Lowers Body Temperature in Rhesus Monkeys Consistent with a Postulated Anti-Aging Mechanism in Rodents," *Proceedings of the National Academy of Sciences of the USA* 93/9 (1996): 4159–64; M. A. Lane et al., "Dehydroepiandrosterone Sulfate: A Biomarker of Primate Aging Slowed by Calorie Restriction," *Journal of Clinical Endocrinology and Metabolism* 82/7 (1997): 2093–96; R. B. Verdery et al., "Caloric Restriction Increases HDL2 Levels in Rhesus Monkeys (*Macaca mulatta*)," *American Journal of Physiology* 273/4 (pt. 1, 1997): E714–19.

9. M. H. Ross, "Length of Life and Caloric Intake," *American Journal of Clinical Nutrition* 25 (1972): 834–38.

10. R. L. Walford, S. B. Harris, and M. W. Gunion, "The Calorically Restricted, Low-Fat, Nutrient Dense Diet in Biosphere 2 Significantly Lowers Blood Glucose, Total White Cell Count, Cholesterol, and Blood Pressure in Humans," *Proceedings of the National Academy of Sciences of the USA* 89 (1992): 11533–37; Roy L. Walford, M.D., and Lisa Walford, *The Anti-Aging Plan: Strategies and Recipes for Extending Your Healthy Years* (New York: Four Walls Eight Windows, 1994); R. L. Walford, L. J. Weber, and S. Panov, "Caloric Restriction and Aging As Viewed from Biosphere 2," *Receptor* 5 (1995): 29–33; R. L. Walford et al., "Biospheric Medicine As Viewed from the Two-Year First Closure of Biosphere 2," *Aviation, Space, and Environmental Medicine* 67/7 (1996): 609–17.

11. G. Fernandes et al., "Dietary Lipids and Calorie Restriction Affect Mammary Tumor Incidence and Gene Expression in Mouse Mammary Tumor Virus/v-Ha—ras Transgenic Mice," *Proceedings of the National Academy of Sciences of the USA* 92/14 (1995): 6494–98.

12. Maren Beth et al., "Comparison between the Effects of Dietary Fat Level and of Calorie Intake on Methylnitrosourea-Induced Mammary Carcinogenesis in Female SD Rats," *International Journal of Cancer* 39 (1987): 737–44; David Kritchevsky, Maxine M. Weber, and David M. Klurfeld, "Dietary Fat versus Caloric Content in Initiation and Promotion of 7,12-Dimethylbenz(a)anthracene-induced Mammary Tumorigenesis in Rats," *Cancer Research* 44 (1984): 3174–77.

13. Z. Huang et al., "Dual Effects of Weight and Weight Gain on Breast Cancer Risk," *Journal of the American Medical Association* 278/17 (1997): 1407–11.

14. Lane et al., "Diet Restriction in Rhesus Monkeys"; Lane et al., "Calorie Restriction Lowers Body Temperature in Rhesus Monkeys"; Lane et al., "Dehydroepiandrosterone Sulfate"; Verdery et al., "Caloric Restriction Increases HDL2 Levels."

15. Intersalt Cooperative Research Group, "Intersalt: An International Study of Electrolyte Excretion and Blood Pressure; Results for 24-Hour Urinary Sodium and Potassium Excretion," *British Medical Journal* 297 (1988): 319–28; Michael Tuck et al., "The Effect of Weight Reduction on Blood Pressure, Plasma Renin Activity, and Plasma Aldosterone Levels in Obese Patients," *New England Journal of Medicine* (April 16, 1981): 930–33; Victor Stevens et al., "Weight Loss Intervention in Phase 1 of the Trials of Hypertension Prevention," *Archives of Internal Medicine* 153 (1993): 849–58.

16. P. K. Whelton et al., "Sodium Reduction in Weight Loss in the Treatment of Hypertension in Older Persons: A Randomized, Controlled Trial of Nonpharmacologic Interventions in the Elderly (TONE)," *Journal of the American Medical Association* 279/11 (1998): 839–46.

17. *New England Journal of Medicine* 332 (1995): 621.

18. Steven N. Blair, "Evidence for Success of Exercise in Weight Loss and Control," *Annals of Internal Medicine* 119/7 (pt. 2, 1993): 702–6; Martha Skender et al., "Comparison of 2-Year Weight Loss Trends in Behavioral Treatments of Obesity: Diet, Exercise and Combination Interventions," *Journal of the American Dietetic Association* 96/4 (1996): 342–46.

19. K. N. Pavlou, S. Krey, and W. P. Steffee, "Exercise as an Adjunct to Weight Loss and Maintenance in Moderately Obese Subjects," *American Journal of Clinical Nutrition* 49 (1989): 1115–23.

20. Kathleen J. Melanson et al., "Fat Oxidation in Response to Four Graded Energy Challenges in Younger and Older Women," *American Journal of Clinical Nutrition* 66 (1997): 860–66.

21. Doris Lennon et al., "Diet and Exercise Training Effects on Resting Metabolic Rate," *International Journal of Obesity and Related Metabolic Disorders* 9 (1985): 39–47.

22. M. A. Flynn et al., "Aging in Humans: A Continuous 20-Year Study of Physiologic and Dietary Parameters," *Journal of the American College of Nutrition* 11/6 (1992): 660–72; E. T. Poehlman et al., "Physiological Predictors of Increasing Total and Central Adiposity in Aging Women and Men," *Archives of Internal Medicine* 155 (1995): 2443–48; S. B. Roberts et al., "What Are the Dietary Energy Needs of Older Adults?" *International Journal of Obesity and Related Metabolic Disorders* 16/12 (1992): 969–76; S. B. Roberts et al., "Influence of Age on Energy Requirements," *American Journal of Clinical Nutrition* 62/5 (suppl., 1995): 1053S–58S; M. Visser et al., "Energy Cost of Physical Activities in Healthy Elderly Women," *Metabolism Clinical and*

Experimental 44/8 (1995): 1046–51; David F. Williamson, "Descriptive Epidemiology of Body Weight and Weight Change in U.S. Adults," *Annals of Internal Medicine* 119/7 (pt. 2, 1993): 646–49.

23. Katch and McArdle, *Introduction to Nutrition, Exercise, and Health.*

24. John P. Foreyt and G. Ken Goodrick, "Evidence for Success of Behavior Modification in Weight Loss and Control," *Annals of Internal Medicine* 119/7 (pt. 2, 1993): 698–701; Skender et al., "Comparison of 2-Year Weight Loss Trends."

25. Nelson and Hekmat, "Promoting Healthy Nutritional Habits."

26. P. M. Dubbert and G. T. Wilson, "Goal-Setting and Spouse Involvement in the Treatment of Obesity," *Behavioral Research and Therapy* 22 (1984): 227–42; W. Hartman, D. Wapner, and J. Saxton, "A Simple Procedure to Identify Persons at Risk for Dieting Failure," paper presented at 24th Annual Conference, Association for Advancement of Behavior Therapy, San Francisco, California, 1990; S. Kayman, W. Brovold, and J. S. Stern, "Maintenance and Relapse after Weight Loss in Women; Behavioral Aspects," *American Journal of Clinical Nutrition* 52 (1990): 800–807; M. G. Perri et al., "Effect of Length of Treatment on Weight Loss," *Journal of Consulting and Clinical Psychology* 57 (1989): 450–52.

27. S. J. Curry, A. R. Kristal, and D. J. Bowen, "An Application of the Stage Model of Behavior Change to Dietary Fat Reduction," *Health Education Reviews* 7 (1992): 97–105; Karen Glanz et al., "Stages of Change in Adopting Healthy Diets: Fat, Fiber, and Correlates of Nutrient Intake," *Health Education Quarterly* 21/4 (1994): 499–519; S. R. Rossi et al., "A Comparison of Four Stages of Change Algorithms for Dietary Fat Reduction," paper presented at the Society for Behavioral Medicine Annual Meetings, San Francisco, California, March 1993.

28. Katch and McArdle, *Introduction to Nutrition, Exercise, and Health,* 223.

29. Two studies presented at American College of Sports Medicine Meeting, May 1997.

30. Barbara E. Ainsworth et al., "Compendium of Physical Activities: Classification of Energy Costs of Human Physical Activities," *Medicine and Science in Sports and Exercise* 25 (1993): 71.

31. Lawrence J. Appel et al., "A Clinical Trial of the Effects of Dietary Patterns on Blood Pressure," *New England Journal of Medicine* 336/16 (1997).

32. J. Rodin, "Environmental Factors in Obesity," *Psychiatric Clinics of North America* 1 (1978): 581–92.

33. Ainsworth et al., "Compendium of Physical Activities."

34. Bidoli et al. "Food Consumption and Cancer of the Colon and Rectum in North-Eastern Italy," *International Journal of Cancer* 50 (1992): 223–29.

35. Appel et al., "A Clinical Trial of the Effects of Dietary Patterns."

36. Jayne Hurley and Bonnie Liebman, "Inside Sandwiches," *Nutrition Action Healthletter* 22/3 (1995): 1+.

37. Briefel et al., "Total Energy Intake of the U.S. Population."

38. Ainsworth et al., "Compendium of Physical Activities."

39. Karen H. Duncan, Jane A. Bacon, and Roland L. Weinsier, "The Effects of High and Low Energy Density Diets on Satiety, Energy Intake, and Eating Time of Obese and Non-Obese Subjects," *American Journal of Clinical Nutrition* 37 (1983): 763–67.

40. David S. Siscovik et al., "Dietary Intake and Cell Membrane Levels of Long-Chain n-3 Polyunsaturated Fatty Acids and the Risk of Primary Cardiac Arrest," *Journal of the American Medical Association* 274/17 (1995): 1363–67; Christine M. Alberts et al., "Fish Consumption and Risk of Sudden Cardiac Death," *Journal of the American Medical Association* 279 (1998): 23–28.

41. D. G. Schlundt, T. Sbrocco, and C. Bell, "Identification of High-Risk Situations in a Behavioral Weight Loss Program: Application of a Disease Prevention Model," *International Journal of Obesity and Related Metabolic Disorders* 13 (1989): 223–34.

42. Duncan et al., "The Effects of High and Low Energy Density Diets."

43. M. Ito and M. Oyama, "Relative Sensitivity to Reinforcer Amount and Delay in a Self-Control Choice Situation," *Journal of Experimental Animal Behavior* 66/2 (1996): 219–29.

ACKNOWLEDGMENTS

Thank you . . .

To my parents. Your love and support give me strength and courage every day.

To my sister, Andi. Two spirits couldn't have a stronger bond.

To my brother-in-law, Stuart, for putting up with all of us.

To Elizabeth Miles, for being in tune with my thoughts. Your passion and tireless work on this book will always be remembered.

To Marcy Posner, my agent and dear friend—you are simply the best!

To my editor, Mitchell Ivers: my heartfelt appreciation for your enthusiasm and vision in sharing portion savvy with the world.

To Liz Hartman, Emily Bestler, and everyone at Pocket Books.

To Jane Temple, for your excellent research, your time, and your patience.

To David Lust, who helps me juggle everything without dropping a ball.

To the many visionary scientists, including Dr. Clyde McKay, Dr. Morris Ross, and Dr. Roy Walford, who have pioneered our understanding of the portion savvy imperative. And a special thanks to Dr. David Levey.

To the Diet Designs staff, for helping me give my clients health and happiness.

To my Diet Designs clients, for proving that portion savvy works day in and day out.

My special thanks to JoAnn Cianciulli, Christy Bray, and Mario Alvarez for your assistance with recipe testing and your devotion to me, Diet Designs, and making a healthy difference in so many lives.

INDEX